Migraine

As many as one in ten people suffer from attacks of migraine, often becoming completely incapacitated. These attacks may involve severe and extremely painful headaches, often localized in one half of the head, and accompanied by nausea and vomiting. The pain may be so severe that the sufferer's faculties are seriously impaired.

Most sufferers are women, whose families are often disrupted during the attacks, as the victim may have to stay completely quiet in a darkened room for a full day or even more. Although the condition has been known for over 1800 years, the cause is still unknown. However, as the author shows, many factors which produce attacks have recently been studied, giving us new knowledge of the trigger factors, particularly diet, tension, depression, water retention, and menstruation.

This book will be welcomed by sufferers and their families. Dr. Hanington explains for example how to handle patients in an attack and how to take preventive measures. The forms of treatment, many of them quite new, are also set out in detail, in the hope of bringing relief to many.

Migraine

Edda Hanington MD

TECHNOMIC PUBLISHING COMPANY

Copyright © 1973 by Edda Hanington
Published in 1976 by
Technomic Publishing Company, Inc.
Westport, Connecticut
Printed and bound in Great Britain by
The Garden City Press Limited
Letchworth, Hertfordshire SG6 1JS
LCC: 76-11273
ISBN: 0-87762-108-5

This book is dedicated to my dear husband, John.

Acknowledgements

I am grateful to my son John for his help with this book and to Mr. Keith Kilby for the line drawings.

Contents

7

What is Migraine?

"Is there anything whereof it may be said, See, this is new?
"... and there is nothing new under the sun".
BOOK OF ECCLESIASTES

THREE and a half thousand years ago another writer was concentrating on migraine. It is mentioned in the oldest medical manuscript known to man. This is the Ebers papyrus which was found in a tomb at Thebes in the middle of the nineteenth century. George Ebers edited the papyrus in 1874. He was born in Berlin in 1837 and studied law, oriental languages and archaeology. After holding a post as Reader in Egyptian language and antiquities at the University of Jena he became a Professor at Leipzig in 1870 and remained there for almost twenty years. He made many journeys to Egypt and was keen on rousing the interest of the public in his own country in antiquities, archaeology and Egyptian history. He decided that the best way to do this was by incorporating these themes into historical romances, which proved to have a considerable appeal. Ebers died in 1898.

In the Ebers papyrus migraine is mentioned as "a sickness of half the head." A description of migraine is also included in the oldest written language in existence. It was during the fourth and third millennia before the birth of Christ that the foundations of the world's first true civilization were laid by the Sumerians in Mesopotamia. It was also at this time that writing was invented as a means of communication. In an extract from the Sumerian account of the Deluge we read about a vision of heaven :

The sick eyed says not "I am sick eyed,"
The sick headed (says) not "I am sick headed."

Ages old though they are these two descriptions give us a very clear account of migraine as we know it today. They tell us that the headache affects one half of the head and that it is accompanied by eye signs and sickness. If we add that it recurs at intervals and frequently runs in families then we have the whole picture.

Migraine was described by the Greek physician Galen who lived from A.D. 130 to 200. Galen was the greatest anatomist and physiologist of classical times and ranked highest as a brain and nerve anatomist. He was born at Pergamum and was surgeon to the gladiators there. He later became physician to the Emperor Marcus Aurelius and was the first to feel the pulse as an aid to diagnosis. He was a careful observer and a prolific writer. Of migraine he said :

> Hemicrania is a painful disorder affecting approximately one half of the head, either the right or the left side, and which extends along the length of the longitudinal suture.... It is caused by the ascent of vapours, either excessive in amount, or too hot, or too cold.

Galen was the founder of experimental physiology. After he introduced the term hemicrania it was gradually modified through hemigrania, emigranea, migranea, megrim to its present form migraine.

Many centuries later John Fothergill who lived from 1712 to 1780 gave a classical description of migraine. Dr. Fothergill, a quaker, became one of the first physicians of his age, although he declined an appointment as a Royal physician. The son of a prosperous farmer of Wensleydale in Yorkshire, he studied medicine in Edinburgh. After receiving his degree he went to St. Thomas' Hospital in London where his kindness and concern for poor patients won him their affection and respect. In later years he is said to have remarked, "I climbed on the backs of the poor to the pockets of the rich." Fothergill was a man who devoted his life to the public good. He was a friend of John Howard, the prisoners' friend, and used his influence to improve the conditions in jails. He was one of the first to install public baths and to effect other sanitary measures. Franklin said of Fothergill, "I can hardly conceive that a better man has ever existed."

John Fothergill read a paper on migraine on 14th December, 1778, entitled *"Remarks on the complaint commonly known under the name of the Sick Headache."* He wrote in this paper,

What is Migraine?

There is a disease, which, though it occurs very frequently, has not yet obtained a place in the systematic catalogues. It is commonly to be met with in practice, and is described by those who are affected with it, and who are not few in number, under the compound title of a sick head ache.

Under this title they, at least, describe their feelings and, on a little inquiry, one finds that they are affected by both. This is not the complaint of any particular age, or sex, or constitution, or season, it is incident to all. The sedentary, inactive, relaxed and incautious respecting diet, are the most exposed to it; and who are yet, sometimes, not much less sufferers by the means frequently made use of to remove it, than by the disease itself.

To collect into a short compass all the symptoms which accompany this disease, would be difficult, and not so very interesting, to describe so many, as to make the complaint easily to be distinguished in the first place, and in what manner it may be treated with success, will be of more importance.

These who are affected with the sick headache, most commonly describe it in the manner; that they awake early in the morning with a headache, which seldom affects the whole head, but one particular part of it, most commonly the forehead, over one frequently, sometimes above both eyes. Sometimes it is fixed about the upper part of the parietal bone, of one side only; sometimes, and infrequently the occiput is the part affected. Sometimes it darts from one to another of these places. It never goes entirely off, from the time it commences, till it wholly ceases, but is sometimes less tolerable.

With this is joined more or less of sickness, and which is just barely, in many people, not sufficient, without assistance, to provoke vomiting. If this pain does happen, as it most commonly comes on early in the morning, and before any meal is taken, seldom anything is thrown up but thin phlegm, unless the straining is severe, when some bitter or acid bile is brought up. In this case, the disease begins soon to abate, leaving a soreness about the head, a squeamishness at the stomach, and a general uneasiness, which induces the sick to wish for repose. Perhaps, after a short sleep, they recover perfectly well, only a little debilitated by their sufferings.

In 1886 about 100 years later Hilton Fagge wrote of migraine :

I do not know of any other malady which within the present (nineteenth) century has been the subject of two papers admitted into the Philosophical Transactions, as well as of communications to the Philosophical magazine and other scientific publications in this country and abroad.

When so much attention was paid to the subject of migraine by eminent men, many of whom suffered from it themselves, it is hardly surprising that it came to be regarded as a disorder affecting the more intelligent. The incidence of migraine is thought to be around eight per cent in the general population. This figure is not, however, spread uniformly throughout life. Migraine is rare in childhood. At five years the incidence is only one per cent or less. By eleven years it has risen to about five per cent in both sexes although the figure varies according to where the survey is taken. At all events the incidence of migraine rises sharply in girls during the teenage years and in the early twenties.

We all know what we mean by headache but surprisingly enough roughly half the population rarely or never suffer from a headache. Approximately one in five of those who do suffer can be classed as migraine subjects. It is, however, difficult to obtain accurate figures for the incidence of migraine. The reasons for this are manifold. To begin with there are a number of people who suffer from headaches but do not recognize that the condition they suffer from is migraine. Perhaps a true story will illustrate this point. During a hunt for volunteers for a migraine research project a nurse was discovered sitting in Sister's office with her head in her hands. She looked up and the pallor of her face was immediately evident. With a harassed expression, she rushed out of the office to return again several minutes later. She confided that she had been very sick and added, "It's my head you know, the pain is all over this side and I feel terrible. I've had these heads since I was small but I'm thankful I don't get migraine." This nurse, who was genuinely amazed when she realized that she did indeed suffer from migraine, subsequently felt much better when she was properly treated. She also took part in the research project!

Migraine had always seemed something very special in the way of headaches to her and this attitude is not uncommon. You will hear people say that they are "feeling bilious," or "It's my liver again." On closer enquiry it is apparent that although the headaches recur at intervals sometimes with other symptoms these people are unaware of the fact that they are migraine sufferers.

A large number of migraine sufferers never consult a doctor about their headaches. They have come to accept them as part of their way of life and the thought of going to the doctor about them does not occur to them. This attitude may of course change with the increasing number of migraine clinics which are being started at present.

To many sufferers migraine is a disorder which they would rather keep to themselves. They are faintly ashamed of their headaches and feel that they are evidence of some sort of personal failure. Furthermore migraine implies a recurring disability. It is obvious that if an employee is forced to take a day off work because of a headache he may well prefer to call it a chill. A vague feeling of guilt often adds to the patient's distress during an attack as it has probably been hinted to him on more than one occasion that if he really made an effort and pulled himself together he would not suffer from headaches. These factors are all somewhat nebulous but nevertheless they indicate some of the reasons why it is difficult to obtain accurate figures for the incidence of migraine.

Added to this the diagnosis of migraine is not always straight-forward. Migraine is not a condition like arthritis or anaemia where definite physical signs in the body indicate the presence of the disorder. In fact if physical signs of any sort were found one might hesitate to make a diagnosis of migraine. These are only a few of the difficulties which arise when one attempts to assess the incidence of migraine in a population.

We can define migraine as a headache, usually affecting chiefly one side of the head, which recurs at intervals. It is often associated with nausea and vomiting. Migraine has been classi-fied into two groups, common migraine and classical migraine. The description of common migraine has already been given and it is about twice as common as classical migraine. In classical migraine the symptoms of unilateral headache, nausea and vomiting are preceded by premonitory signs called an aura. These signs are a warning and herald an attack. They are usually followed by the onset of headache within a period of approximately fifteen minutes. The signs are usually visual and they vary from one patient to another although they remain fairly constant to the individual person.

One patient may see zigzag lines. These are called fortification spectra and may form bizarre shapes. Another patient will see flashing lights while a third will notice that a part of his field of vision has been blotted out. This loss of part of a visual field is called a scotoma. In much rarer instances temporary paralysis of a limb or even of one half of the body may herald an attack. In a very few patients no headache follows these premonitory symptoms but in the greater majority they are followed by the onset of one sided head pain.

It is difficult to give an exact figure for the incidence of classical migraine. About half of migraine sufferers experience classical attacks at one time or another, but the number of patients who get classical symptoms every time they suffer from a headache is probably much lower and in the region of ten to fifteen per cent.

In some migraine sufferers the onset of an attack is preceded by a feeling of extra well-being, excess energy, or hunger. Individual patients get to know their own warning signs and to act accordingly. Vast tomes have been written about the auras of migraine but no useful purpose would be served by digressing on them here.

The pain in migraine is felt mainly on one side of the head. Usually patients say that one side is affected far more often than the other, but that pain has on occasions been felt on either side. The most common areas where pain is felt are around the eye and temple, on the side of the head, or spreading up from the back of the neck over the top of the head.

The pain in migraine varies in severity, from one attack to another in the same patient, and from one patient to another. It is a sickly, throbbing pain aggravated by any kind of stimulus such as a bright light, movement, noise, exertion or straining. The pain increases in intensity over a period of one or two to several hours and then gradually fades away. Patients also describe shooting and stabbing pains through the head during an attack. After a severe attack of migraine has passed the affected side of the head often feels sore for a day or two and as though the pain would start again with the least provocation.

A patient in the throes of a migraine attack usually looks cold and pale. The face appears pinched and the hands and feet are cold. One of the most unpleasant features of migraine is the intense nausea and vomiting which often accompany the headache. In a small proportion of patients diarrhoea may also occur. You may never have had an attack of migraine but if you were ever extremely sea sick and wished that the boat would sink, then remember what that felt like. Add a pounding headache to those symptoms and you will have some idea of how a sufferer feels in an acute migraine attack.

Migraine is familial, that is it tends to run in families. About sixty per cent of migraine sufferers report that other members of their family suffer from migraine but careful studies have shown that its incidence in the families of migraine sufferers is over ninety per cent. More than half of the migraine sufferers questioned report that one or other of their parents suffer or suffered from migraine. Mothers are more often responsible for the inheritance of migraine than fathers. Sceptics have suggested that the incidence of migraine is familial because children grow up observing and imitating their elders. This, however, is unlikely as only one child in a family of three children may become a migraine sufferer and psychological studies have not revealed any traits that might lead to this difference.

Migraine attacks tend to occur in cycles. If a headache is constantly present it is not migraine, as the intervals between attacks of migraine should be free of headaches. The free intervals may vary from a day or two to several months and subjects are usually aware of the fact that they have phases when almost anything will start off a headache. At other times they are far less liable to develop an attack. Furthermore there is a refractory period after an attack when they are highly unlikely to get a headache even if the factors which usually produce one are operating.

It used to be thought that migraine sufferers were particularly intelligent. This suggested in a delicate and consoling manner that the headaches were the price one paid for extra brain power. The thought may have comforted many a sufferer or at least made him feel a member of a privileged community, but the facts do not confirm the theory.

Common and classical migraines are the two types of headache which commonly occur. But before we go on to consider the other variants of migraine we must consider the subject of tension headache.

TENSION HEADACHE

A headache which is constantly present is more likely to be a tension headache than migraine. This type of headache usually affects both sides of the head and patients often describe it as a weight on the head or a tight band around the head. Investigations have shown that about half the patients who attend neurological clinics because of their headaches are suffering from tension headache. As its name suggests it is often associated with stress and worry. This causes a tightening in the muscles of the head and neck and tenderness on pressure is often felt in the muscles at the back of the neck and at the base of the skull. The main differences between tension headache and migraine are its site, the fact that it may be present more or less constantly and the character of the pain. We all know people who have a chronic headache and look permanently harassed. There are border line cases, however, where tension headache merges into migraine. The dull, persistent pain of tension headache then changes to the localized severe, throbbing pain of migraine. This switch over from tension headache to migraine occurs in about one in ten sufferers from tension headache They are the patients who have typical attacks of migraine at intervals but who state that they are never really free from pain.

CLUSTER HEADACHE

Cluster headache, as its name suggests, occurs in clusters or batches. It affects men more often than women and usually starts in adult life between the ages of thirty and forty years. It has, however, been known to begin in the early twenties.

The headache is severe, throbbing in character and felt on one side of the head, usually in the region of the eye. It may spread as far as the lower jaw or around the ear. The pain is abrupt in onset, lasts for a brief period from a few minutes to about two or three hours and then fades away. The pain may recur once or several times a day for a period ranging from two or three weeks to two or three months. There may then be long intervals varying from months to years when the individual is free from pain. The affected side of the face may become very flushed during an attack of cluster headache, and it may be associated with severe watering of the eyes, especially the eye on the affected side of the head. The nostril on the affected side may also feel blocked.

A family history of headache is not typical in cluster headache as it is in migraine, although migraine appears to be somewhat more common in the first degree relatives of sufferers with cluster headache than in the general population. Cluster headache does not usually have the warning symptoms frequently associated with the onset of a migraine attack.

It appears very likely that the sensitivity of the blood vessels in the affected area is altered in patients with cluster headache during the period when attacks occur. This is of great interest as provoking factors can induce an attack during the time when the vessels are sensitive whereas they will have no effect at all at another time. For example, patients who are suffering from a bout of cluster headaches will develop an attack within thirty to fifty minutes after taking a tablet containing one milligram of nitroglycerine under the tongue. Again a substance called histamine which is poured out in the tissues in response to shock, injury or an allergic reaction will in small doses induce an attack of cluster headache in a sufferer during a susceptible period. At other times neither nitroglycerin nor histamine will have any effect. In any case one has to leave a latent period of about eight hours from the last attack before attempting to induce a second one by any means. Alcohol is another substance to which the sufferers from cluster headache are very sensitive during headache spells. At such times it should be strictly avoided. The onset of a bout of cluster headaches appears to be related to a rise in the histamine levels in the blood. It has been noticed that when patients who suffer from angina also suffer from cluster headache their anginal symptoms often improve during a bout of headaches.

Cluster headaches do not usually respond to treatment with ergot in the way that typical migraine attacks often do. Antihistamine drugs by mouth are sometimes helpful.

One of the biochemical changes which is typical of the onset of a migraine attack does not occur in cluster headache. This is the fall in the blood of serotonin, but this will be dealt with at greater length in the section dealing with biochemical changes. There is another point of interest which differentiates a migraine attack from cluster headache. The human eye resembles a balloon filled with liquid. Changes in pressure in the fluid in the eye occur with every pulse beat and these changes can be measured and recorded. In patients suffering from cluster headache a marked increase in the amplitude of pressure changes occurs during an attack of pain. No such increase has been found in patients suffering from an ordinary migraine attack.

Treatment of cluster headache has sometimes been attempted by histamine desensitization. A histamine base has been given daily in doses starting at 25 µg and rising by increments of 5 µg daily to a dose of 100 µg. This level is maintained for three weeks and then reduced to a maintenance dose of 100 µg per week. The role of histamine will be mentioned again in the section of this book dealing with biochemical changes.

MIGRAINOUS NEURALGIA

In some patients who suffer from migraine the character of their headaches changes with the passing of the years. The typical headaches which they used to have are replaced by episodes of neuralgic pain. This may affect the ear or the cheek and usually occurs on one side of the head only.

OPHTHALMIC MIGRAINE

This is a rare form of migraine in which the disturbances of vision which can herald an attack of classical migraine are encountered without any headache. The patients who suffer from this often consult an eye specialist because of sudden, alarming loss of vision. This may be accompanied by flashing lights or zigzag lines. This transient loss of vision usually occurs in an older age group of patients and is restricted to one eye, but the symptoms can occur in younger people and usually last for a very short while only.

Another type of migraine, which is somewhat similar, in so far as disturbances of vision occur, is also found among young people, mainly young women. Apart from the visual symptoms, giddiness is felt and the patient becomes unsteady, talks indistinctly and develops a severe headache in the back of the neck. This type of migraine is very rare.

In ophthalmoplegic migraine, which is also very uncommon,

paralysis of one or more of the eye muscles occurs with a uni-lateral headache.

All these more alarming types of migraine are extremely rare. Fortunately migraine is not a fatal disorder, but obviously expert advice should always be obtained when any of these rare types of migraine occur.

We have considered the subject of tension headache and seen how it differs from migraine. There is another type of headache which is sometimes confused with migraine and which should be mentioned here.

TEMPORAL ARTERITIS

Temporal arteritis is a condition that occurs in an older age group of patients. It usually affects people over the age of sixty-five but can occur at any time from about fifty years to eighty years. Like migraine the condition is paroxysmal but the pain of temporal arteritis often affects both sides of the head. It may vary in its position and in its severity but can occur in the jaw, scalp, tongue or neck. Ordinary analgesic remedies such as aspirin and codeine do not relieve the pain.

If you put your finger on the side of your face just in front of your ear you will feel the temporal artery beating. In patients suffering from temporal arteritis this artery may become tender to touch. In addition it becomes thickened and tortuous, and the normal pulsation is no longer felt. Areas of tenderness may also develop on the scalp.

The vital point about temporal arteritis is that medical atten-tion should be sought immediately. A number of patients with this disorder develop eye symptoms within four weeks of the onset of symptoms and it is essential to treat the condition at an early stage if permanent disturbances of sight are to be avoided. Patients with temporal arteritis generally look and feel unwell. Whereas the typical migraine sufferer feels fit between attacks the sufferer from temporal arteritis often suffers from anaemia and loss of weight and may be feverish.

If a small section of the temporal artery is examined typical pathological changes are seen in this condition which again makes it different from migraine where intensive searching has failed to reveal any characteristic pathological changes in the affected blood vessels. The patient with temporal arteritis should be treated in hospital as soon as the condition is diagnosed.

TRIGEMINAL NEURALGIA

Another paroxysmal condition which has to be differentiated from migraine is trigeminal neuralgia. This is a rare condition which can occur late in life and gets its name from the trigeminal nerve, one of twelve nerves arising directly from the brain rather than the spinal cord. Sensation from the face is transmitted in the sensory fibres of the trigeminal nerve and occasionally a very painful neuralgia develops in this nerve. The attacks are paroxysmal and acutely painful as can be seen from the description of a patient given by Dr. J. Waring Curran over 100 years ago.

> During our conversation a paroxysm commenced. In the middle of a remark, like a flash of lightning, the pain set in, truly pitiable to observe; he was unable to complete his sentence and could only tell me that the left side of the head felt "as if" he said, "it was being chipped with a butcher's hatchet." I gathered that the pain was worst within the head, spreading with lessened severity to the peripheral termination of the nerves. Truly his agony was great, and as I was informed it would continue two hours at least, I tried if possible to relieve him, sending for some chloroform and liniment of aconite, which I painted along the course of the affected nerves.

The treatment has changed in the past century, but the pain of trigeminal neuralgia remains one of the most severe forms of suffering.

2

Other Causes of Headache

> "Then you should say what you mean" the March Hare went on.
> "I do," Alice hastily replied; "at least, at least I mean what I say,
> that's the same thing, you know."
> "Not the same thing a bit!" said the Hatter.
> —Lewis Carroll. *Alice's Adventures in Wonderland*

IF we define a headache as a pain in the head then we mean
what we say. But if the Mad Hatter could appear to tell us that
this is not the same thing at all as saying what we mean then we
would have to agree with him. But let me explain before it all
becomes too complicated.

The causes of pain in the head are legion. They range from
such conditions as toothache and earache to eye strain and sinus
trouble. None of us would really consider any of these types of
headache as the sort of thing that we refer to when we talk about
a headache, although one could not deny that a pain in the head
is present in all these states. Perhaps we could leave the likes of
Alice and the March Hare and the Mad Hatter to sort out the
technicalities of the matter and concentrate on the causes of what
we really mean by a headache.

Volume for volume the head is the heaviest part of the body.
The weight of the head is reduced a little by virtue of the fact
that it contains a number of air pockets or sinuses. When a sinus
becomes infected, which can happen in such conditions as a
heavy cold, the membrane lining the wall of the affected sinus or
sinuses becomes inflamed. It may become so inflamed that fluid
oozes out and a fluid level may then be seen on an X-ray
picture. Inflamed sinuses are one of the possible causes of
localized pain in the head.

The bones of the head can be separated into the skull which

contains the brain and the bones of the face. The skull forms a solid case protecting the brain which is a relatively soft organ. The brain is wrapped in three tissue paper-like sheaths and cushioned by a thin layer of fluid (cerebrospinal fluid) which circulates between them. This fluid acts as a buffer between the brain and the spinal cord on the one hand and the bones of the skull and backbone which provide a solid frame for them. The cerebrospinal fluid acts as a shock absorber and its composition and pressure are regulated by a very delicate mechanism.

Because the skull is rigid the space within it is strictly limited. Pain arises when any change occurs in the pressure within the skull. Such a change in pressure may result from changes in the volume of cerebrospinal fluid. In a condition like meningitis the volume of fluid increases and headache occurs. In a lumbar puncture a few drops of cerebrospinal fluid are removed by means of a small hollow needle which is inserted between the third and fourth lumbar vertebrae in the spine. When the volume of cerebrospinal fluid increases it is found to be under increased pressure when a lumbar puncture is done. Occasionally a lumbar puncture investigation, which involves drawing off a small quantity of cerebrospinal fluid through a hollow needle, is followed by a headache because of a fall in the pressure of the fluid. A change in pressure can also result from traction or pull on the blood vessels within the skull. This can result from inflammation, from injury, from changes in pressure of the cerebrospinal fluid or on very rare occasions from the expansion of such things as abscesses within the skull. Even minor alterations in the size of blood vessels within the skull produce pain, and this is the commonest cause of headache. Dilation of the arteries within the skull occurs from a number of causes and the resulting headaches are called vasodilator headaches. They can be recognized by their characteristic features. They are throbbing in character and the pain affects both sides of the head. It becomes worse with any jerking or jarring such as stooping or lifting. This type of headache results from a large number of causes ranging from an ordinary hangover to climbing at high altitudes. Vasodilator headache also occurs in fevers and as a result of the injection of foreign protein as in vaccination.

The headache associated with high blood pressure usually arises in older people. It affects the back of the head and is present first thing in the morning when the sufferer wakes up. It wears off rapidly when the patient gets up and moves around. Taking too many analgesic tablets is a cause of headache which probably occurs more often than is recognized. Patients who overdose themselves with pain killing drugs may set up a constant cycle of headaches. The subject of rebound headaches due to drug therapy is mentioned again in the section of this book on drug treatment.

As there is so little room for expansion inside the skull it is relatively easy to understand why headache occurs when the blood vessels within the skull dilate. It is more difficult to grasp why headache occurs when blood vessels on the outside of the skull, where there is plenty of space, increase in size. In a migraine attack the blood vessels on the outside of the skull are affected. The branches of the external carotid artery on the painful side of the head become enlarged. An interesting fact, which may or may not be relevant to the pain in migraine is worth noting. The external carotid artery sends branches through perforations in the skull into the area within the skull on the side of the head and to the bony socket of the eye. These are two of the most common sites of pain in a migraine attack. It is difficult to see how one could find out for certain, but it is just possible that distension of these vessels running from the outside to the inside of the skull is partly responsible for the pain which is present in migraine. We know that biochemical changes occur around the affected blood vessels in an attack of migraine and that these changes are linked with the production of pain. The fact that branches from these affected vessels run from the outside of the head to the interior of the skull may be an added factor in pain production.

The condition of trigeminal neuralgia has already been mentioned in the section describing migraine. Nerve pain affects the area supplied by the nerve. Typically brief attacks of severe pain occur in a localized area.

Pain is not always felt at its site of origin. For example, pain due to an abscess under the diaphragm may be felt in the shoulder. This is because sensations from the diaphragm and the shoulder are transmitted by nerves which both arise from the same segment of the spinal cord. When the impulses of sensation are transmitted the pain may be referred from one area to the other. Roughly speaking the fifth cranial nerve transmits sensation from the front two thirds of the head and the first three nerves running from the spinal cord transmit sensation from the posterior third of the head. The fibres of the nerves seem to overlap somewhat and for this reason disorders of the neck may occasionally result in headache and neck pain may also sometimes occur with headache.

3

What Happens in a Migraine Attack?

BEFORE an illness develops there is often a period of time when the individual does not really feel well. Later on, when the illness manifests itself we frequently hear the patient say "Oh, that must be why I wasn't feeling too good in the past few days." It may even be a relief to the sufferer to find that something positive is wrong with him because now this can be treated in the proper way.

The opposite state of affairs is true for some migraine sufferers. For some hours before the onset of an attack they feel extra well, cheerful and full of energy. It is rather unfortunate that they gradually come to recognize that this burst of good spirits is a warning of trouble ahead in a very literal way! Other migraine sufferers feel ravenously hungry before an attack, while others keep yawning or have the feeling that they are growing larger in size or smaller than usual. Of course these sensations do not affect every migraine sufferer but they occur sufficiently often to be worth mentioning. Undoubtedly they are associated with biochemical changes which occur at the onset of a migraine attack and which result in changes of mood.

One of the greatest physicians of the seventeenth century was Thomas Willis. He was described as a plain man, of no carriage and little conversation, but despite this he was appointed as physician to the King. Willis had great powers of clinical observation and was the first person to notice the sweetish taste of diabetic urine. This was, of course, long before the time when chemical tests were employed to detect sugar in urine. At one time Willis was the Sedleian Professor of Natural Philosophy in Oxford but in 1667 he moved to London and began to practise. It was said of him that "never any physician before went beyond him or got more money yearly than he." Willis died in 1675 and is buried in Westminster Abbey.

Willis is of interest to us for two reasons. He was the first to describe the arterial circulation at the base of the brain. This is still known by the name of the circle of Willis. Secondly Willis has left us a graphic account of the headache history of a famous Society letter writer of her day, Lady Anne Finch Conway, who lived between the years 1631 and 1678. Lady Conway suffered severely from migraine and was attended by a galaxy of illustrious physicians of that time in her attempts to obtain relief from this affliction. Thomas Willis was one of them and described her distressing symptoms in the following words:

A certain noble Lady (whose sickness is below described) for the curing of a cruel and continual Headache, underwent a plentiful Salivation three times, viz., the first by a Mercurial Oyntment, by the consel of Sir Theodore Mayern, and afterwards twice by taking the lately famous Powder of Charles Huis, without any help, I wish not with some detriment : for afterwards for many years, even to this day, the disease being by degrees increased, she suffered under its heavy tyranny.

Some years since, I was sent for to visit a most noble Lady, for about twenty years sick with almost a continual Headache, at first intermitting. She was of a most beautiful form, and great wit, so that she was skilled in the Liberal Arts, and in all sorts of Literature, beyond the conditions of her sex; and as if it were thought too much by Nature, for her to enjoy so great endowments, without some detriments, she was extremely punished with this Disease. Growing well of a Feavour before she was twelve years old, she became obnoxious to pains in the Head, which were wont to arise, sometimes of their own accord, and more often upon every light occasion. This sickness being limited to no one place of the Head, troubled her sometimes on one side, sometimes on the other, and often thorow the whole compass of the Head. During the fit (which rarely ended under a day and a night's space, and often held for two, three, or four days) she was impatient of light, speaking, noise, or of any motion; sitting upright in Bed, the Chamber made dark, she would talk to no body, nor take any sleep, or sustenance. At length about the declination of the fit, she was wont to lye down with an heavy and disturbed sleep, from which awakening, she found herself better, and so by degrees grew better, and continued indifferently well till the time of the intermission. Formerly, the fits, came not but occasionally, and seldom under twenty days or a month, but afterwards they came more often; and lately, she was seldom free. Moreover, upon sundry occasions or evident causes (such as change of the Air, or the year, the great aspects of the Sun and Moon, violent passions, and errors in diet), she was more cruely tormented with them. But although this Distemper grievously afflicting this noble Lady, above twenty years (when I saw her) having pitched the tents near the confines of the Brain, had so long besieged its regal tower, yet it has not taken it; for the sick lady, being free from a Vertigo, swimming in the Head, Convulsive Distempers, and any Soporiferious symptom, found the chief faculties of her soul sound enough.

For the obtaining a Cure, or rather for a tryal, verymany Remedies were administered, thorow the whole progress of the Disease, by the most skilful Physicians, both of our own Nation and the prescriptions of others beyond the Seas, without any success or ease; also great Remedies of every form and kind she tryed, but still in vain. Some years before, she had endured from an oyntment of Quicksilver, a long and troublesome Salivation, so that she ran the hazard of her life. Afterwards twice a Cure was attempted, (though in vain) by a Flux at the mouth, from a Mercurial Powder, which the noted Empirick Charles Hues ordinarily gave; with the like success with the rest she tryed the Baths, and Spawwaters almost every kind and nature; she admitted of frequent Blood-letting, and also once the opening of an Artery; she had also made about her several issues, sometimes in the hinder part of her Head, and sometimes in the forepart, and in other parts.

She also took the air of several Countries, besides her own Native Air, she went to Ireland and into France. There was no kind of Medicines, both Cephalicks, Antiscorbuticks, Hysterical, all famous Specifics, which she took not, both from the Learned and unlearned, from Quacks, and old Women; and yet notwithstanding, she professed, tho she had received from no Remedy, or method of Curing, anything of Cure or Ease, but that the contumacious and rebellious Disease refused to be tamed, being deaf to the charms of every Medicine. Further, this so long possessing the out-parts of the Head, though it could not invade the cloisters of the Brain; yet when I visited her, unfolding its ends in some other parts of the nervous kind, it had begun to stir up most cruel pains in her members and also in her Loins, and bottom of her Belly, as is wont to be in the Rheumatism, and in the Scorbutick Colic.

Poor Lady Anne Conway. As Thomas Willis writes at the end of his treatise on her complaint,

For from any other cause, if there had been a conflict of Nature's Medicine with the Disease, either a quick death or a joyful Victory had far sooner been attained.

We know that migraine is a vascular disorder and that changes occur in the affected blood vessels during an attack. The organs of the body obtain the food and oxygen they require through the blood stream. Blood is carried to all our organs by arteries, and most organs are adequately supplied with blood through one main artery. The arteries are paired when the organs are paired like the kidneys. The brain and the heart are both well protected from damage, lying as they do within the framework of the skull and rib cage. The brain is unique, because it is supplied by no less than three main arteries. These are the two carotid arteries and the basilar artery.

The carotid arteries can be felt, and sometimes seen beating on either side of the neck. Each of the carotid arteries divides into an internal carotid branch which runs into the inside of the skull and an external carotid artery which supplies blood chiefly on the outside of the skull. Running up the backbone, on either side of the spinal cord are the vertebral arteries. The vertebral arteries join together at the base of the skull to form the single basilar artery. The basilar artery joins with branches from the two internal carotid arteries to form a highly efficient arterial circuit at the base of the brain. This arterial circuit, first described by Thomas Willis is known as the circle of Willis and is shown in Figure 1. It ensures that even if one part of the blood supply to the brain is blocked for any reason the brain will still receive an adequate blood supply through the rest of the circuit.

Outside the skull or cranium, that is on the outside of the head, the blood supply is provided by the external carotid artery on each side of the head.

ARTERIES AT THE BASE OF THE BRAIN
THE CIRCLE OF WILLIS

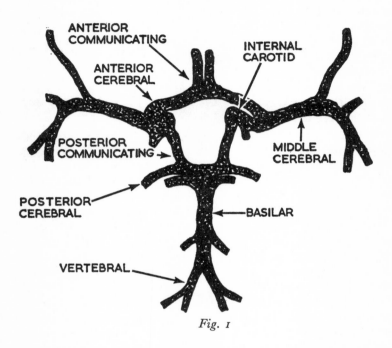

Fig. 1

The blood supply inside the skull is called the cerebral circulation and the blood supply on the outer side of the skull is called the extracerebral circulation.

It is obviously essential that the centres of the brain which control vital functions in the body such as the heart beat and breathing should receive an adequate blood supply. Nerve cells have no stores of glucose like the cells in muscles to call upon in an emergency. They are dependent on the nutrients carried to them by the blood. Oxygen is essential to the life of cells in the human body and this too is carried in the red cells of the blood.

The striking feature about the blood supply to the brain is the extremely delicate way in which it is controlled. This regulatory mechanism acts in a completely independent way to the control of the circulation in the rest of the body. This is hardly surprising when one considers the functions of the brain and the fact that it is contained within the rigid casing of the skull. If every time we sat in a hot bath we dilated the blood vessels supplying our brains it might produce some strange effects quite apart from a headache. The delicate mechanism which controls the blood flow to the brain ensures that the brain cells receive a constant oxygen supply and an adequate supply of essential nutrients.

It seems likely that most people who suffer from migraine are born with a constitutional tendency for their blood vessels to react in an abnormal way to certain stimuli. This tendency can also be acquired through the action of certain drugs. On the whole most sufferers from migraine have a family history of headache and this constitutional factor is present. Superimposed on this constitutional tendency are trigger factors which actually precipitate a headache. These are many and various and range from such things as exposure to cold, extreme fatigue and eating chocolate.

Migraine is a vascular disorder, which means that it is a disorder of blood vessels. Vascular headaches have certain recognizable features. These are chiefly the character of the pain which throbs with every heart beat. Any physical effort exacerbates the pain. Such acts as lifting up a suitcase may greatly increase the severity of the pain and bending down to pick up something from the floor may change it from being severe to becoming almost unbearable. In a severe attack of migraine even raising the head from a pillow may increase its pounding. Similarly coughing increases the pain. The only way in which the pain can be alleviated a little without drugs is by the sufferer lying completely still with the affected side of the head buried in a pillow. This produces some degree of pressure on the affected vessels and gives a little relief.

Three stages are recognized in a migraine attack. During the first phase there is a narrowing of the branches of the carotid blood vessels. This narrowing affects the vessels on both sides of the head and not only the vessels on the side that becomes painful. How do we know this? There are various methods that one can use to see what is going on in blood vessels, such as injecting a substance which is opaque to X-rays into the blood stream. This substance shows up on an X-ray picture and outlines the contours of the vessels. This has been done during the prodromal phase of migraine and narrowing of the vessels has been shown.

The only way in which blood vessels can be viewed directly in the intact body is by means of an instrument called an ophthalmoscope. With this instrument a light is shone through the pupil on to the back of the eye which can then be inspected through a magnifying lens. What is seen when one looks through an ophthalmoscope is shown in Figure 2. At the back of the eye is the retina which is the part of the eye sensitive to light. Across the retina are the fine terminal branches of the optic nerve which transmits the impulses from the retina to the centres in the brain which are responsible for interpreting vision. The head of the optic nerve is seen as a flat white disc, the optic disc, on the retina. Across the retina runs a network of arteries and veins, and by examining these one can obtain a good idea of the general state of the blood vessels in the body. For example in a patient with a high blood pressure changes occur at an early stage in

THE VIEW THROUGH AN OPHTHALMOSCOPE

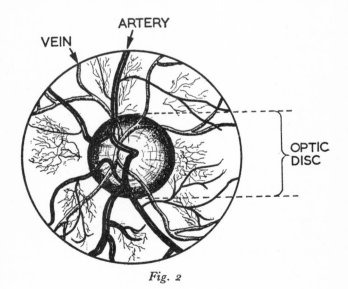

Fig. 2

THE ARTERIES OF THE SCALP
BRANCHES OF THE EXTERNAL
CAROTID ARTERY.
(shaded areas indicate sites of pain in migraine)

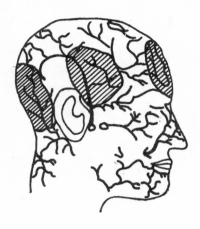

the blood vessels of the retina. Changes are found in some patients with diabetes and in a large number of other disorders. Thus an examination of the retina with an ophthalmoscope is a routine part of a medical examination.

The blood vessels on the retina have been observed during the prodromal stage of a migraine attack. This is the time during which the sufferer from classical migraine complains of warning symptoms such as visual disturbances already described. Examination of the eyes with an ophthalmoscope has confirmed that during this phase the retinal vessels on both sides of the head become narrowed. In fact the blood flow in the internal carotid artery may be reduced to half its previous level.

The blood vessels in the cerebral circulation are extremely sensitive to changes in the oxygen and carbon dioxide content of the blood. A rise in carbon dioxide levels causes a dilation of the cerebral blood vessels. It is interesting to note that the prodromal symptoms of migraine are sometimes relieved when the

Fig. 3

sufferer breathes in and out of a paper bag. This simple measure increases the carbon dioxide content of the blood and causes the cerebral vessels to dilate.

The prodromal phase of migraine during which constriction of the vessels takes place is followed by a stage in which the vessels on the side of the head on which pain develops become enlarged and throbbing. The vessels affected at this stage are the branches of the external carotid artery and these dilated, throbbing branches can often be seen standing out on the side of the head in the painful area (see Figure 3).

Changes in the amount of blood flowing through a vessel can be measured by the technique of thermography. Whenever an area becomes inflamed the blood flow to that site increases. This produces heat, and heat is one of the four cardinal signs of inflammation. Pain, swelling and redness are the other three signs. One has only to think of the hot, red, swollen painful area surrounding a boil or carbuncle.

Thermography is a technique which can be used to record heat radiation from the surface of the body. It is possible to obtain a visual record of this heat production and this is called a thermogram. Tumour tissue for example emits more heat than normal tissue and thermography is being used in order to detect very early cases of cancer of the breast. Mass screening of women has been undertaken in some parts of the country but the method is time consuming and has to be repeated at intervals. It is still in a state of trial and whether or not it will eventually prove to be a universally applicable method of investigation remains to be seen.

Serial thermography has been undertaken in the various stages of a migraine attack. This has demonstrated the changes in blood flow associated with the different stages of an attack of migraine.

The fact that the blood flow is increased in the painful area of the head during the headache phase may lead you to wonder why the migraine sufferer so often looks pale during an attack. After all an increased blood flow should produce heat and redness. It is highly likely that shunts occur between the arteries and veins in this area so that despite the fact that more blood is flowing through the arteries it is rapidly shunted off into the veins without passing through the capillary bed. Vessels directly

· ·

linking arteries and veins through which such shunting could occur are known to be present.

The pain of migraine cannot be due solely to the dilation of blood vessels in the affected area. These vessels dilate in a similar way whenever one sits in a really hot bath for a while. And fortunately migraine sufferers do not get migraine because they enjoy a hot bath. Why does pain occur around the dilated vessels in migraine? The vascular changes appear to result in response to chemical changes which take place in the body of a migraine sufferer during an attack. The biochemical techniques required to carry out research into these chemical changes have only become available in recent years and a great deal of interest is now concentrated in this field. As yet the changes resulting in pain in migraine are poorly understood but they are dealt with further in another section of this book.

4

The Causes of Migraine

TIRESOME children, blood pressure, tension at work, lack of sleep, too much to drink—all are commonly cited reasons for the headaches we wake up with or go to bed with. We all like to blame something for our aches and pains even if it is only that unfailing scapegoat, the weather. But are the reasons that we so readily find really to blame? Can such things as getting harassed, missing meals, drinking a bit too much alcohol or having a slightly raised blood pressure be responsible for headaches?

In June 1972 the Office of Health Economics produced a booklet on migraine. This was a factual statement on the subject and among the information given was a list of trigger factors which could precipitate an attack in a susceptible individual. This list of triggering factors is alarming in its length and is as follows :

Anxiety
Worry
Emotion
Depression
Shock
Excitement
Overexertion
Physical and mental fatigue
Bending or stooping as in gardening
Lifting heavy weights or straining of any sort
Changes of routine, e.g. holidays, shift work or change of job
Late rising, especially at weekends or on holiday
Travel
Change of climate
Changes in weather—high winds
Bright sunlight, bright artificial light or glare of any kind, fluorescent light
Prolonged focusing on television or cinema screen
Very hot baths
Noise, particularly loud and high pitched sounds
Intense odours or penetrating smells
Certain foods, e.g. fried foods, chocolate, citrus fruits, pastry and cheese
Use of sleeping tablets
Alcohol
Prolonged lack of food—fasting or dieting
Irregular meals
Menstruation and the pre-menstrual period
Menopause
High blood pressure
Continued use of oral contraceptives
Toothache and other local pains in head or neck

This list was originally produced in *Focus on Migraine* (1971) published by The Migraine Trust.

When such opposite reasons as eating too much and eating too little, or sleeping too much and sleeping too little can all result in a headache, it is small wonder that the fundamental cause of migraine has remained obscure.

Let us read what Henry Handford, Physician to the General Hospital in Nottingham, had to say in 1898 about the causes of migraine.

I must omit many things entirely, and confine myself chiefly to my own views, and to the description of a few phenomena which appear to me to have attracted little or no attention. And this is the most remarkable, for as Gowers says, the disease is often associated with high intellectual ability, and many distinguished scientific men have suffered from it, and have supplied more careful observations of the subjective symptoms than we possess of any other malady. Among the sufferers may be mentioned the celebrated Dr. Fothergill, Marmontel, Haller, Wollaston, du Bois-Reymond, Sir Charles Wheatstone, Sir John Herschell, Sir George Airy, his son Dr. Hubert Airy and our present President of the Royal College of Physicians, Sir Samuel Wilks. From this you may gather that, however painful and temporarily disabling migraine may be, it is not incompatible with a long life and a vast amount of work of the very highest quality.

Migraine is strongly hereditary. Usually paroxysmal headache will be found to have occurred in an ancestor or some member of the family. Frequently only a general neurosis is inherited, one member of the family suffering from one form of nervous disease and one from another. The most frequent nervous "associations" are neuralgia, epilepsy, chorea, gout. This shows that whatever view of the intimate pathology be accepted, a nervous substratum is almost invariable.

Where there is no faulty inheritance it will commonly be found that the nervous system has been brought into a state of imperfect nutrition, either by losses of blood, by want of sufficient fresh air and exercise, by sustained intellectual exertion, or by some exhausting disease.

The chief exciting causes are worry, fatigue, excitement, impure air, cold, or indiscretions of diet, the latter acting either alone, or more commonly in association with one of the preceding causes. In many people the combination of the fatigue of a railway journey with an unusually long interval without food, and followed by a substantial meal, will almost certainly cause an attack; whereas none of these conditions acting singly is sufficient. In some very susceptible patients, chiefly women, a railway journey alone is sufficient. The general vibration, and the effect upon the eyes of quickly passing objects, seem to be as important as the mere fatigue; and these are generally associated with either cold or close impure air, both of them important causes of migraine.

Migraine

In speaking of digestive disturbances as a cause of an attack, Gowers writes "Frequently, after the usual interval between the attacks has nearly elapsed, a slight error in diet is sufficient, although soon after the patient has had an attack even actual indigestion has no effect."

Another frequent cause, which hardly receives the attention it deserves, is cold. It acts both by inducing indigestion, and also probably by depressing the nervous centres and leading to vasomotor changes.

In those with a gouty or rheumatic tendency or inheritance, alcohol, especially in the form of the imperfectly fermented wines, such as champagne, is a fertile source of attacks.

In some people running brings on an attack, suggesting that disturbance of the circulation may be the immediate exciting cause. The degree of the exciting cause required to produce an attack varies immensely, and inversely with the robustness of the patient.

I know one patient, a lady of about forty-five, of highly artistic tastes, who has lived chiefly in large towns, and taken very little out-of-door exercise, in whom a visit to the theatre or to a concert is generally followed by one or two days prostrating migraine. No doubt the close poisonous atmosphere plays as important a part as the fatigue and excitement, especially in producing vasomotor changes.

Another patient, subject to attacks every two or three months, married at the age of forty. After about a year, a child was born, and for the next eighteen months she devoted herself entirely to the care of her child, never going away from home, being very little out of doors, (half an hour to one hour daily), and gradually drifting into a very anaemic condition, with marked impairment of the general health. The reason of my being asked to see her was that the attacks now came on every two or three weeks instead of months, and the one in which I saw her had already lasted seven or eight days, and was causing alarm from its persistence. The two special causes here were the impaired general health and cold. She was one of those people who do not keep their rooms and houses sufficiently warm. But such people often suffer severely from cold in the form of impaired digestion, diarrhoea and generally depressed vitality. Too much of their energy is used up in maintaining body heat.

This diversity of cause has been one of the reasons why the subject of migraine has remained a mystery for so long. But let us return to our own list at the beginning of the chapter and look at the causes that people commonly blame for their symptoms

Let us take blood pressure first. This is one of the less likely

36

causes. An abnormally high blood pressure can occasionally be the cause of headaches but this is by no means the rule. The headache of hypertension or high blood pressure is most often present when the individual wakes up in the morning. As soon as he or she gets out of bed and starts moving around the headache usually wears off. Of course the ideal arrangement would be for the hypertensive person to be brought an early morning cup of tea. Then he or she could sit up and enjoy it and get up gradually.

It has been reported that the incidence of migraine is considerably higher in a group of patients with a raised blood pressure than in a matched group of patients with a normal blood pressure. When patients with a raised blood pressure complain of headaches these usually improve when the raised blood pressure is treated, so that a doctor should be consulted.

But what about the others? Are people right to blame their headaches on the fact that they are harassed or that they have eaten or drunk too much or too little? A long list of the possible precipitating factors in migraine has already been given. If we consider the most common causes we could group them as follows :

Stress
Low blood sugar
Dietary factors especially citing
   Chocolate
   Cheese
   Alcohol
Hormonal factors

Most migraine sufferers are aware of a number of factors which can precipitate their attacks. During a good phase of the migraine cycle one may be able to have a late night and take a drink with impunity. During a headache phase even a minor lapse is likely to precipitate an attack of pain.

Migraine runs in families. The sufferer appears to be born with a constitutional predisposition to the disorder. The blood vessels in migraine patients appear to react to certain stimuli in a way that results in headache. It seems that this type of reaction can also be sometimes acquired through the action of various agents such as oral contraceptives.

It appears likely that there is a factor linking all the causes of migraine and that this unifying factor is a disturbance of amine metabolism. In order to understand how and why a disturbance of amine metabolism may affect the body to produce an attack of migraine a brief description of the nervous system is needed.

The functions of the body are controlled in two ways. They are under the control of chemical messengers called hormones. These are secreted into the bloodstream by a number of endocrine glands such as the pituitary gland and the thyroid gland and the concentration of the hormone in the bloodstream controls a variety of activities. The second way in which the actions of the body are controlled and co-ordinated is through the nervous system.

The nervous system consists of two parts. One of these is the central nervous system comprising the brain and spinal cord with the nerves arising from them. It receives sensory impulses and controls voluntary movement. The other, the autonomic nervous system, regulates those functions of which we are unaware and which are completely beyond our conscious control, such as the rate of the heart beat and the movement of the intestine. It is a highly complex system composed of two parts, the sympathetic and the parasympathetic. The actions of these two parts are opposite in effect, for example the sympathetic fibres dilate the pupil and cause an increase in the rate of the heart beat. Stimulation of the parasympathetic fibres constricts the pupils and slows the heart rate.

One of the main functions of the sympathetic nervous system is to control the size of blood vessels. The actions of the autonomic nervous system are brought about by chemical means. There are two chemical transmitters in the autonomic nervous system, namely acetylcholine and noradrenaline. The chemical which is usually released at the ends of sympathetic nerve fibres is noradrenaline which, like adrenaline, belongs to a group of substances called catecholamines. The catecholamines are produced in the body in two ways. Under certain conditions they are secreted by the suprarenal glands, which are small glands situated just above the kidneys. They are also released at the ends of sympathetic nerve fibres where they supply organs such as blood vessels. When the catecholamines are released by the suprarenal glands they augment the effect of stimulation of the sympathetic nervous system.

And what sort of conditions result in the release of catecholamines? They are briefly listed as follows:

Any state of stress
Low blood sugar which occurs with hunger or starvation
Dietary factors especially the intake of alcohol
Overexertion
Hormonal factors

Has anything struck you about this list? If not please read and consider it again. You probably saw the link straight away. All the conditions which lead to a change in catecholamine metabolism are also conditions which can result in a migraine attack.

Migraine is a vascular disorder in which changes occur in blood vessels. Blood vessels are regulated by the action of the sympathetic nervous system, which is mediated by the chemical transmitter noradrenaline, one of the catecholamines. Little by little we can see how the pieces of the jigsaw could gradually fit together. We have a rough idea of what the whole picture is about when we appreciate the fact that the conditions which are associated with an alteration in catecholamine metabolism are the same conditions that can lead to the onset of an attack of migraine.

If we consider migraine in this way then I think that we can begin to see the link between the various causes. They all start a similar chain of events in the body resulting in a common chemical end point which produces an alteration in blood vessel size and pain in the affected area. We have to find out why, in identical circumstances, one person is prostrated by an attack of migraine while another is headache free. It is not enough to say that there is a constitutional difference, which is usually hereditary, between the sufferer and the non-sufferer. We want to know what this difference is and as more investigatory techniques become available the problem should eventually be solved.

The need for more research into migraine is obvious. But even if we find the answers we are seeking there is no guarantee that they will provide new solutions to the problem as far as practical measures for the individual sufferer are concerned.

It would be unwise to wait for the results of further research in the hope that they will provide a magic formula to banish migraine completely. We should take advantage of all the knowledge we already have available and migraine sufferers should consider carefully and do something about these factors in their own lives which could be contributing to their attacks.

Other points of interest arise when we think about the causes of migraine. For example one migraine sufferer may have frequent attacks while another rarely has a headache. It is not unreasonable to suggest that the person with infrequent attacks reacts less readily to the various possible precipitating factors. This individual variation applies to every aspect of human physiology and behaviour. Sometimes migraine attacks begin to occur for the first time in an older person. If this should happen it is important for the sufferer to obtain medical advice. In women these headaches of late onset are sometimes associated with the hormonal changes that occur at the time of the menopause.

Many of the factors that lead to headaches in adults also play a role in the headaches of childhood. In the words of Wordsworth, himself a sufferer from severe migraine, the child is father of the man. Causes such as hunger, fatigue and dietary factors are relatively easy to identify in children, but stress which is such a common cause of migraine attacks may be much more difficult. Children can become very worried over matters to which no adult would give a second thought and considerable perception may be needed to discern them. For example a child may find reading difficult and become so anxious on a day when he thinks that he might be asked to read aloud at school that a headache develops.

The essential point to emphasize is that migraine is a condition in which many factors can play a precipitating role. When more than one is present, for example when a woman gets overtired and misses a meal just before a menstrual period (three possible precipitating causes) a headache is far more likely to develop than if only a single factor were concerned.

Before leaving the causes of migraine we can take note of the advice of Dr. John Fothergill who published his rules for the preservation of health over two hundred years ago. He said that these came into being as the result of many years of practice. The word distemper is somewhat outmoded today but doubtless we shall all see what he means when he writes

> When distempers are perceived to make their approach they should be prevented by removing their causes as soon as possible. A man seems to be in a middle state between health and sickness, when he has some slight ailment that does not confine him to his bed or from his business, such as an inconsiderable headache, loss of appetite, some unusual weariness, weight or drowsiness, but it is the part of a wise man to prevent these small disorders from growing worse, by correcting without delay the disposition from which they are derived. If, for example, the complaint arises from too great a fulness, that fulness should be diminished by abstinence or (if abstinence is not sufficient) by bleeding, purging or sweating.

On 4th May, 1662, Samuel Pepys wrote in his diary :

> Mr. Holliard come to me, and let me blood, about sixteen ounces, I being exceedingly full of blood and very good. I begun to be sick; but lying upon my back I was presently well again, and did give him 5s for his pains ... after dinner, my arm tied up with a black ribbon, I walked with my wife to my brother Tom's.

No doubt Samuel Pepys could write equally sanguinely about purging and sweating. Fortunately for us these somewhat drastic measures have passed from our armentarium of treatment. In considering the distempers of today, such as migraine, our approach to the problem is altogether less harsh. Nevertheless we can all profit from the general advice of the physicians of that time such as John Fothergill. Without the investigatory aids available to doctors now they were forced to rely on their own powers of acute observation, and the lessons of experience. Experience after all remains the greatest personal teacher, and experience teaches the migraine sufferer that his best line of treatment is moderation in all things.

YOU AND YOUR MIGRAINE

You may be interested in the subject of migraine in general, but if you are a sufferer then what you really want to know is what you can do about it.

On one of the walls of the most famous temple to Apollo at Delphi in ancient Greece the words "Know thyself" were inscribed. At first sight this might seem a sound and relatively simple precept to follow but how difficult it proves to be in practice. To be honest with ourselves is far from easy.

One of the first tasks that every migraine sufferer should set himself is trying to find out why his attacks occur when they do. It is useless throwing your arms in the air and saying that you have no idea why you get headaches and how on earth could anyone expect you to know. One thing is certain, if you do not attempt to find out yourself, then no one else can. So where does one begin? We can start by taking another look at the most common causes of migraine. These are

Stress
Hormonal factors
Dietary factors
Low blood sugar

Stress covers a wide field of precipitating causes ranging from the excitement of a visit to the theatre to the anxiety of wondering whether or not the gas tap was turned off at the oven.

Probably the easiest way to discover why your migraine attacks occur when they do is by keeping a record of them over a period of time. A minimum period of at least three months is advisable. If you have a pocket diary it is easy to jot down when you get a headache and to note any associated factors that could have played a part in causing it. Women should record the dates of menstrual periods as the hormonal cycle so often bears a relation to the incidence of headache. This fact may not be immediately apparent. Headaches often occur midway between two monthly periods, and it is only when a careful record is kept that the link gradually becomes evident. A note should also be made of any possible dietary factors that could be relevant, such as the eating of chocolate or the taking of alcoholic drinks. Similarly you should note if you missed a meal or if any other circumstances arose that might have contributed to your headache. Only you can know what these factors might be as they vary so much from one person to another.

Stress is often unavoidable. If you know that a situation that will upset you is inevitable then it is only sensible to see whether you can prevent a headache from occurring by taking precautionary measures. Making an effort to prepare in advance may prevent the last minute rush which so often precipitates a headache. It may be worth taking a mild sedative tablet or an extra Dixarit tablet or even a long acting aspirin tablet. It may sound ridiculous to treat yourself in advance but if you consider it logically a little preventive therapy wisely applied may prove a far better investment than having to take far more potent therapy a little later on when a headache develops.

There are a number of relatively simple points that every migraine sufferer should observe apart from the more obvious ones that have already been noted. For example, it is hardly surprising if you end up with an attack of migraine if you spend an hour or two heaving heavy furniture around, when you are not accustomed to this form of exertion.

We are all individuals and migraine sufferers must remember that it is only as individuals that they can hope to work out what the contributing causes to their headaches may be. For example, constipation or the taking of excessive laxatives can both be aggravating factors during a spell of recurring headaches.

The next few sections of this book will be dealing with the specific causes of migraine and how one might seek to remedy them. Clearly it is only possible to deal with the more common causes of migraine. Even if you do not feel that your particular case falls into any of the descriptions given, on reflection you will probably find that it is closer than you imagined. For example, someone may be muttering "Ah, but I always get a headache when I drive on the motorway with all those glaring headlamps, and that cause of migraine hasn't been mentioned anywhere. And it must be a fairly common cause because they are always writing about it in the newspapers." So it may be! But if you think about it you will probably agree that you hate the glaring lights and find this particular type of driving a great strain. Could you deny that if driving in these circumstances worries you the stress involved in such a journey is probably considerable?

The needs of children who suffer from migraine are not dealt with separately. Many of the factors which can precipitate migraine in adult life can also operate in childhood. The application of common sense will point to the practical measures which should be taken. These are often so much easier to carry out when you are looking after someone else than when you are taking care of yourself.

5

Pain

PAIN is like the red light at the traffic signals. It pulls us up with a jerk. It forces us to pause and to take stock of the position. Although many a migraine sufferer would agree with John Dryden when he comments

> "For all the happiness mankind can gain
> Is not in pleasure, but in rest from pain."

none would deny that pain serves an essential purpose in making us aware that all is not well with our bodies. There are some rare conditions in which the sensation of pain is lost. When this occurs extreme care has to be taken by the individual to compensate for this loss of sensation. For example if an eye becomes anaesthetic particles of dust will get into it causing damage and ulceration which could lead to blindness. If fingers or toes lose their feeling they will easily be burned or crushed. It is obvious therefore that pain serves an essential function in our bodies.

When we are well it is difficult to imagine what pain feels like. Let us hope, however, that we do not confirm Samuel Johnson's observation that "those who do not feel pain seldom think that it is felt." The degree of pain felt by another person is naturally difficult to assess. If someone is writhing around with

44

severe colic we are all aware of the fact that he is in great pain. But there are many chronic conditions, such as rheumatoid arthritis, where the sufferer may have to put up with a considerable degree of pain with nothing dramatic to show for it. We all tend to be sympathetic to the person who has an accident or an acute illness but when a state of ill health is prolonged it is easy to forget the suffering borne by the afflicted person.

The word pain is derived from the Latin word "poena." The Latin word is translated as penalty or retribution and in primitive societies pain was often regarded as a punishment from the gods. Pain is usually associated with inflammation. The classical description of inflammation was given by Celsus, a Roman nobleman, who lived at the time of Christ. Celsus was a follower of Hippocrates the father of medicine and he wrote books on philosophy, military science, agriculture, law and medicine. Only the book on medicine is still in existence and was first printed in Florence in 1476. Celsus describes inflammation by four signs, calor, rubor, tumor, dolor—heat, redness, swelling and pain.

The pain threshold is the level at which pain is felt. This varies from one person to another. If a person is in good health and feels fit he is able to tolerate pain better than a person who is tired, overanxious and run down. On the whole children have a higher pain threshold than adults. How many adults would be covered in smiles like the cheerful schoolboy with cuts and bruises all over his legs? A method has been found for measuring the pain threshold and one can see how this threshold differs between one person and another. One way of measuring the pain threshold of a person is by applying pressure with a thin tube over the mastoid process or bump just behind the lobe of the ear. The pressure required to produce the beginnings of a painful sensation varies from half a kilogram to six kilograms per square centimetre, but the majority of people feel pain with a pressure of about two kilograms. Surprisingly enough, women tend to feel pain at a lower threshold than men!

Pain is transmitted through the nerve endings in the skin and internal organs. The factors which produce pain differ in different parts of the body. For example if you cut through the skin it is painful, but if you cut across your intestine, if it were possible to do such a thing without damaging anything else, you would not feel pain. Your lungs distend with air with every breath and it is painless but severe flatulence can be very painful. You can sit in a hot bath and dilate all the blood vessels in your skin, and end up looking as red as a tomato and it will not be painful. But if you dilate the blood vessels inside your skull even to a minor degree it will cause pain. The muscles of the legs contract without pain but contractions of the muscles of the womb can produce pain. Thus the causes and types of pain differ in different parts of the body.

If any migraine sufferers were asked what they considered to be the chief symptom of their migraine attacks they would probably reply that it is pain. In an attack of migraine the arteries in the painful area of the head become enlarged and can often be seen throbbing and pulsating. They are often tender on pressure and the areas around them feel boggy and swollen. The threshold for deep pain is lowered in the painful area which means that less pressure is needed to produce pain in these tissues during a headache period than when the patient is headache free. The pain in migraine usually starts as a throbbing pain. It may gradually increase until it becomes a constant severe ache. The pain is usually localized to an area of the head which is typical for the individual but it may extend to the face, eyes or neck. The pain is made worse by any movement or any type of physical strain.

A lot of interesting work has been done in attempts to discover how pain is produced and why it occurs. In some of this research a cantharidin plaster has been applied to a small area of smooth skin such as the forearm, about one centimetre in diameter. The plaster is left on overnight and by the next morning a blister will have formed. The fluid in this blister is gently sucked out with a small needle and syringe and the dead skin of the blister is carefully cut away. This leaves the raw area at the base of the blister exposed. Normal saline, which is salt solution made up to the same strength as the salt solution contained in the blood, causes no pain when applied to this raw area. The area is, however, highly sensitive to chemical irritants. If the blister fluid which was sucked out of the blister is kept in a glass tube for an hour and then dropped back on to the raw blister severe pain results. Why should this occur when the fluid previously protected the raw area and caused no pain? The interesting fact is that during the hour that the blister fluid was kept in the glass tube a substance developed in the blister fluid responsible for producing the severe pain when the fluid is reapplied. The blister fluid consists of plasma containing protein. Contact with glass activates this protein and breaks it down. A pain producing substance called bradykinin is produced. Normal blood consists of red blood cells, white blood cells and the fluid plasma. Plasma contains a group of substances called kinins and these are associated with the production of pain. The best known kinins are bradykinin and kallidin. If pure bradykinin is applied to the blister bases even in minute concentrations it can provoke pain. The pain produced by bradykinin usually rises gradually to a peak which is maintained for a time before subsiding. It also produces pain when it is injected under intact skin or into an artery. When a minute dose is injected into the carotid artery it produces severe pain along the branches of the external carotid artery but the effect differs with the dosage used. At one dosage level intense pain occurs in the head with perhaps temporary partial loss of vision and nausea. If the dose is only one fifth as large, the vessels in the affected area simply dilate and become more permeable. This permeability is characteristic of pain production and is common to all types of inflammation, whether it occurs in the joints as in rheumatoid arthritis or in the head as in migraine. Permeability implies that vessels allow substances that are normally contained in them to diffuse through into the surrounding tissues. All this work on pain production has been carried out in volunteers who have been fully aware of the nature and purpose of the investigation. It is important to emphasize this lest some readers grow anxious and decide that they will never go near a migraine clinic in case anyone tries to experiment on them.

The kinins in the blood which play a major role in the production of pain are formed by the action of a substance called kallikrein. This is found in the pancreas or sweetbread and in saliva and is excreted in urine. Kallikrein is also produced by the action of the enzyme trypsin or proteolitic snake venom on plasma. Some investigations were carried out on volunteers during a migraine attack. A lumbar puncture was done on each of these volunteers and it was found that the enzymes concerned with the production of the pain-producing kinins were increased in the spinal fluid in half the patients investigated. During a migraine attack the vessels in the affected areas of the head are extremely sensitive to much smaller doses of bradykinin than will usually produce pain.

Histamine is another substance that will produce generalized headache even in non-migrainous people if it is injected intravenously in relatively small doses. The headache produced by histamine is usually accompanied by flushing of the face. If histamine is given in this way to a migraine sufferer during an attack it does not cause a generalized headache but greatly increases the pain already present on the affected side of the head. This unilateral pain in migraine has always been very hard to explain, but the fact that a histamine injection produces a generalized headache, unless the subject is a migraine sufferer in the throes of an attack, suggests the relevance of Hippocrates' dictum that "when two pains occur together but not in the same place, the more violent obscures the other." Another point of interest arises on the subject of unilateral pain in migraine. Occasionally the suffering of a migraine patient has been so severe and so localized that attempts have been made to relieve the pain by cutting the nerve supplying the affected area. This, of course, relieves the previous symptom at the expense of producing an insensitive site on the head. The advantages of this might outweigh the disadvantages of severe recurrent headache, but for the fact that after a shorter or longer period the painful migrainous attacks begin to recur on the other side of the head where the nerve supply is intact.

The advent of modern therapy has done a great deal to alleviate some of the pain of migraine sufferers. This was not always the case. Nearly two hundred years ago Thomas Jefferson, who was elected the third President of the United States and inaugurated in 1801, wrote to a friend

> An attack of the periodical headache which came on me about a week ago rendering me unable as yet either to write or read without great pain.

We can all take courage from the fact that his severe recurrent headaches did not prevent him from being the author of the Declaration of Independence.

6

It's All in the Mind

WE know the faith healer from Deal who said

> Although pain isn't real
> When I sit on a pin
> And it punctures my skin
> I dislike what I fancy I feel.

Most of us have met people like him even if they do not come from Deal. One of the most distressing aspects of suffering from migraine is the lack of sympathy which many people, including some doctors, have with this complaint. Seldom being afflicted with headaches themselves they find it difficult to appreciate the problems of those who are.

Most of us are ill at one time or another. One of the advantages of a brief spell of ill health is that it helps one to realize, at least for a while, what chronic illness must be like. Like the faith healer from Deal we find it easier to recognize suffering through our own experience. Why do so many people lack sympathy for migraine sufferers and even regard them as rather a nuisance? Well, first of all the migraine sufferer has little or nothing to show in evidence for his complaint. If you are limping along with your foot in plaster everyone is aware of the fact that you have a disability. But if you are working in an office and have to leave for home, albeit looking a little pale, because your head is pounding, people are quite likely to think that there is not really anything wrong with you and that if you really made an effort you would be all right.

Secondly, migraine attacks are so often associated with a particular chain of events that it is hardly surprising if an unbiased onlooker came to the conclusion that it is "all in the mind." If every time that you are looking forward to a dinner party you spoil the occasion by getting a headache, if junior ruins every picnic by being sick, and if mother is always trying

49

to cope with an attack of migraine as well as the Sunday lunch, what other conclusion could the onlooker draw?

Nobody would attempt to deny the fact that the workings of the mind and body are closely linked. We have only to think of those commonly used expressions, going red with rage and white with fright. Our emotions can produce profound changes in our bodies. Your heart will pound if you get a sudden shock. Emotion has a marked effect on the circulation. The changes that have been mentioned such as changes in skin colour and pounding of the heart are associated with changes occurring in blood vessels. When your face becomes red small blood vessels in your face have temporarily increased in size. When it turns pale they have constricted.

We know that migraine is a disorder of blood vessels. It is hardly surprising, then, that emotional factors which can produce blood vessel changes can also initiate a pattern of response resulting in migraine.

Ah, says the sceptic, just as I thought. It is all in the mind! But this is not really fair as other people also get anxious, angry and frightened without developing migraine. Furthermore emotional stress is only one of the many factors which can precipitate an attack. There are many other causes of migraine, such as hormonal factors, over which the sufferer has no control. It would therefore be unjust to attribute all attacks to emotional factors. It seems that the affected blood vessels in a migraine sufferer are more susceptible to stimuli than those in a non-sufferer and that this inherited constitutional factor causes the migraine sufferer to react in this way. The same pattern of response can be acquired by non-migrainous people when they are treated with certain drugs.

The study of psychology is a rapidly expanding field. As a developing science it is sometimes regarded with suspicion, but it is only through the application of scientific method that we shall be able to relate mental stress and physical behaviour. It may be of interest to those who would like to dismiss migraine as a condition that is "all in the mind" that psychological studies have shown that migraine sufferers cannot be grouped together in any particular psychological category. Even the consoling thought that migraine sufferers are a more intelligent section of the population has had to be abandoned.

While refuting the accusation that migraine is all in the mind we have to accept the fact that psychological events can produce physiological changes in the body which sometimes result in a headache in migraine sufferers. In other individuals a gastric ulcer or a skin rash may be the outward signs of inward stress. Of course one cannot relate all skin rashes, for example, to mental strain and it would be ludicrous to suggest that one could. Nevertheless there are some disorders of which experience teaches us the physical symptoms frequently bear a close relationship to the mental state of the sufferer. These disorders are termed psychosomatic.

Stress is an alarm signal to the body. In response to this warning the body pours out certain hormones or messengers which prepare the body to take action. Two of these hormones are the catecholamines adrenaline and noradrenaline. They are secreted by the suprarenal glands. A great deal of research into migraine points to an alteration in the metabolism of these hormones during an attack. Furthermore, the one factor which seems to be common to all the causes of migraine is an alteration in catecholamine metabolism. The catecholamines have very powerful actions on blood vessels, but all these aspects are dealt with more fully in the section on the causes of migraine. Another hormone which is secreted in increased amount during periods of stress is pitressin. This is produced by the pituitary glands and one of its actions is to cause water to be stored in the body. The retention of body water is associated with the onset of migraine in some patients. More research needs to be undertaken into this aspect of migraine.

Stress can also produce an effect on the body in other ways. People who are under strain tighten up their muscles. This may result in a grim looking face but the taut muscles can also cause pain. Patients with tension headache suffer in this way. Similarly patients with arthritic changes in the bones of the neck frequently hold their heads in a rather rigid way and this can cause muscular tension and pain. Muscular tension can be an added factor in the severity of an attack of migraine.

The extent to which the mind can influence the body is shown by the number of people who think that they feel better when they are treated with placebo therapy. Placebo treatment is the administration of a substance which can have no effect whatever on the patient or the condition being treated. It is sometimes given when clinical trials are undertaken to see whether or not a new line of treatment is effective or not. Obviously any new therapy has to be tested to judge whether or not it is any use before it is put on the market. Either it will need to be tested against another treatment whose value has already been established, or it can be compared with a course of placebo therapy which cannot possibly have any effect at all, other than psychological. When drugs are administered in clinical trials the patients are told that they are taking part in a clinical trial. The therapy which is to be assessed and the placebo therapy are made to look identical so that the person being treated does not know which he is receiving. The results of treatment are carefully assessed statistically and all the relevant factors such as age, sex, severity and duration of the condition being treated are taken into account.

If approximately equal numbers of patients appear to improve under treatment with the new drug which is on trial and the placebo therapy, then it is clear that the drug being tested is not having the desired effect. If, on the other hand, a significantly larger number of patients improve on the new drug then it is probably of therapeutic value. The improvement on placebo therapy in patients with migraine is usually reckoned to be about thirty per cent.

Reserpine is a drug which has sometimes been used to produce an attack of migraine in patients who have volunteered to take part in research into migraine. About seventy-five per cent of migraine sufferers will develop an attack within a few hours of being given a dose of reserpine. If another group of migraine sufferers is given a harmless injection of sterile water about thirty per cent of them will also develop an attack within a few hours. This makes the difficulties of carrying out research into migraine very obvious. For example, a considerable number of migraine sufferers state that they avoid eating chocolate because it gives them a headache. If you try to test the truth of this statement by giving samples of chocolate to one group of volunteers who complain that chocolate affects them and an identical looking placebo sample to another similar group, about thirty per cent of the individuals tested will react with a headache to the placebo sample. This makes it harder to obtain statistically significant results for the chocolate samples as large numbers of people need to be tested to obtain them.

It is easy to scoff, but psychological factors probably operate in all of us in different ways. Fortunately most of us do not develop migraine as a result.

But what can the migraine sufferer do to help him or herself? The first step towards solving a problem is to recognize the fact that it exists. Of course, it would be very helpful if we did not have to live with our particular difficulties. It would be pleasant if the person we find difficult were further removed from us or if we lived somewhere else. Usually, however, we have to accept the fact that we must cope with our surroundings as they are and not as we might wish them to be. It is even more important to accept the fact that we are unlikely to change other people. Our actions may influence other people so that they wish to change themselves but we cannot be the prime movers of such change, as this must come from within. There is only one change that we can try to make with any certainty of success and that is a change in ourselves. It may take time, effort and patience but if we persevere we can succeed.

Let me give you a simple example. No doubt you will consider it too simple to fit your own particular problem, but that may be partly because we are all very good at making molehills out of other people's mountains and doing the opposite with our own worries.

One of my patients was suffering from increasingly severe, recurrent headaches. She was working in a small office which she shared with another woman similarly middle-aged. This patient was a perfectionist, anxious to do all her work as well as possible. Her companion at work was less conscientious and not at all bothered about whether or not she got through her share of the work on one day or the next. My patient tried repeatedly to influence her companion and to make her more aware of their duties as she saw them. It is hardly surprising that she used to spend at least one day a week away from work with a splitting headache. At her stage in life it was useless suggesting that she should find another equally senior job, which in any case might well present snags of its own. The only way in which she could really tackle the problem was by changing her own attitude to it. She gradually came to realize that she was beating her head against a brick wall by trying to alter someone whose outlook on life was so different from her own. Of course, she had to remain as conscientious as ever herself, but equally she had to stop trying to impose her standards on her neighbour. She could console herself with the fact that example is the best teacher and leave it at that. Although the situation may look unchanged to the unseeing eye this patient succeeded to a considerable extent in changing her own attitude to the problem and found life more tolerable as a result. Her headaches, needless to say, improved.

Yes, you may think, that was a very simple problem. My own is much more difficult. Our own problems always are. But there is only one way to tackle them. We must do something positive about them even if the only positive thing we can do is to accept the fact that they exist and that this is the way things are.

Each of us consists of body, mind and spirit. Man does not live by bread alone. For many people life seems to be an incessant struggle against adversity. The basic necessities of life, of which the majority of our fellow men on this earth are deprived, are obviously essential. Beyond this, however, material wealth can provide greater comfort but it cannot ensure contentment. It is only through trying to maintain a sense of proportion in our lives and by reflecting on ultimate values that we can hope to achieve equanimity with both our neighbours and ourselves. In our hectic civilization many of us find little time to pause and meditate but we should all remember that here we have no abiding city and that peace comes from within.

These thoughts are expressed so very much more adequately in the Book of Proverbs.

> Happy the man who findeth wisdom
> And the man who obtaineth understanding!
> For the merchandise of it is better than the merchandise of silver,
> And the gain of it than fine gold.
> More precious is it than pearls,
> And all thou cans't desire is not equal to it.
> Length of days is in her right hand;
> In her left hand are riches and honour.
> Her ways are ways of pleasantness,
> And all her paths are peace.

7

Headache and Hunger

"LET me have men about me that are fat," said Julius Caesar and he must have had his reasons. One of them we are told in Shakespeare's play was that the lean and hungry Cassius seldom smiled.

We all expect a fat man to be jolly. Of course we all know fat people who are miserable. In fact some of us would say that some people become fat because they are miserable and eat to console themselves in the inevitable disappointments of life. But on the whole we expect a fat man to be cheerful. He is round and comfortable and his very size suggests a human failing with which we can readily sympathize and which makes us feel that in return he will take an equally tolerant view of our shortcomings. To put it briefly, we feel at ease with him. But are there, perhaps, physiological reasons for the good humoured approach to life that is his trademark?

One of the cults of western civilization is the modern craze for slimming. We are led to imagine, through advertisements and exhortation that a sylph-like figure will provide the answer to most, if not all, of life's problems! Health, romance and happiness will be ours if we shed those surplus pounds! However alluring the prospect may be, drastic slimming also has its disadvantages and one of them is the irritability that often accompanies chronic hunger. This irritability may of course be less apparent to the slimmer than to his family and friends as it is easy to turn a blind eye to our own faults. It may, however, be more difficult to ignore the tiredness and headaches that can accompany a rapid loss of weight.

We all need energy. Sometimes we have days when we feel full of energy. On other days we are disinclined to do anything and everything is too much of an effort. Energy is more than a vague term that means nothing. We derive our energy from the food that we eat, which provides the fuel that our bodies require to keep running. Starchy food is converted into glucose and this is broken down in the cells of the body to provide energy in the form of heat.

Digestion is the process by which the various foods we eat are broken down by the digestive enzymes or juices into a form which can be absorbed into the bloodstream through the intestinal wall. All carbohydrate or starchy foods such as bread, potatoes, biscuits, cake, sugar and other sweet things are turned into glucose. The digestion of carbohydrate begins in the mouth where a substance in saliva starts breaking down starch. When we eat a starchy meal it takes one to two hours for the carbohydrate to be transformed into glucose and begin to pass into the bloodstream, but if we eat pure glucose the level of glucose in the blood begins to rise within thirty to sixty minutes. In this way pure glucose provides us with a rapid source of energy.

The normal level of glucose in the blood is between eighty and one hundred milligrams per hundred millilitres of blood. If the blood sugar level drops below forty to sixty milligrams per hundred millilitres we will feel weak and trembly and tiredness and headaches may occur. In order to investigate the blood sugar level a glucose tolerance curve is obtained. The patient is fasted overnight. In the morning, before any other food is taken a dose of fifty grams of glucose is given. Small samples of blood are then taken from a vein in the arm at half hourly intervals over a two hour period and the glucose content of these blood samples is estimated. A graph is made plotting the glucose content of the blood against the timing of the samples. This is called the glucose tolerance curve, and examples are shown in Figure 4.

Insulin is essential to glucose metabolism. The glucose level in the blood is regulated by the amount of insulin in the blood. In a healthy person the blood glucose level rises to a level of about one hundred and sixty milligrams in half an hour to an hour after fifty grams of glucose is given orally in a glucose tolerance test. Diabetic subjects suffer from a lack of insulin and because of this much higher blood sugar levels even exceeding three hundred milligrams per millilitre may be reached in a glucose tolerance test. The fasting level of blood glucose is also often

TYPICAL GLUCOSE TOLERANCE CURVES AFTER 50g OF GLUCOSE IS GIVEN.

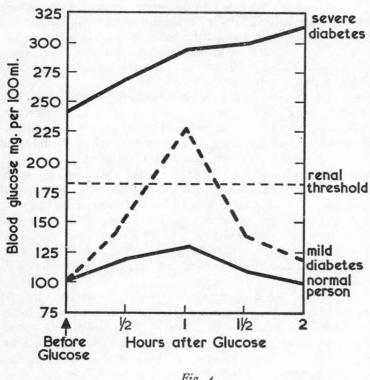

Fig. 4

abnormally high in diabetics. Urine samples are also taken before and during the period of a glucose tolerance test and these are checked for the presence of sugar, not found in the normally healthy person.

The renal threshold level is the blood sugar level at which sugar begins to leak through the kidneys into the urine. The kidneys act as a very delicate filter but sugar does not usually pass from the blood into the urine unless the level in the blood is over one hundred and eighty milligrams per hundred millilitres. Some individuals, however, have a lowered kidney or renal threshold and their kidneys allow sugar to pass from the blood into the urine at a lower blood sugar level. These individuals may have sugar in their urine but a glucose tolerance investigation, which relates the blood sugar level to the sugar present in the urine, shows that their blood sugar levels are within normal limits. Patients with a lowered renal threshold may be losing sugar in the urine but they are not diabetics, since diabetics have raised blood sugar levels. A lowered renal threshold also occurs in some patients during pregnancy.

After it passes into the bloodstream the glucose is dispersed in various ways. Some remains circulating in the body, to provide an immediate source of energy wherever it is required. Some is stored, mainly in the liver, in the form of a substance called glycogen, from which it can readily be converted back into glucose and used for energy if needed. Muscles also store glycogen. Excess glucose, which is not circulating or laid down in glycogen stores, is converted into fat and most of us are well aware of the fat depots in our bodies. When the blood sugar level falls, as in fasting or during heavy exercise, the glycogen is mobilized rapidly and changed back into glucose. In extreme circumstances such as starvation, even fat can be metabolized into energy.

Every cell in the body requires glucose and as has already been explained a large reserve of glucose is stored in the form of glycogen. Nervous tissue, however, contains no glycogen stores on which to call in an emergency and nervous tissue cells have to rely on glucose carried to them in the blood. If the blood sugar level falls sufficiently low, these nerve cells are deprived of their needs and coma and convulsions may occur. The state in which the blood sugar level falls below the normal fasting blood sugar level of eighty milligrams per hundred millilitres is termed hypoglycaemia. This state can occur in such conditions as prolonged fasting, heavy exercise or when a diabetic accidentally has an overdose of insulin.

When the blood sugar level falls some people develop a dull, throbbing headache. Some feel faint and become giddy. This fall in blood sugar occasionally occurs in otherwise fit people who have been eating normally. It sometimes occurs in healthy people between the ages of thirty and forty years, who feel faint, weak and trembly for a short period of time. These symptoms are transient and clear up as soon as a sweet drink is taken.

Some migraine sufferers are liable to develop a headache if they miss a regular meal. In fact volunteers for migraine research have sometimes been asked to fast for a while in order to precipitate an attack. Biochemical studies have then been undertaken both before and during the headache period in an attempt to discover the changes that occur.

Migraine is a disorder of blood vessels. It seems very likely that the nerves which control the size of blood vessels are influenced by changes in blood sugar levels. There certainly appears to be a link between blood sugar levels and migraine. It has been noted, for example, that when diabetic patients suffer from migraine the attacks of migraine tend to occur when their blood sugar levels are low. The opposite also appears to be true as in the rare instances where a migraine sufferer develops diabetes. It has been noticed that the onset of diabetes with its attendant rise in blood sugar levels has been associated with a diminution in the frequency and severity of migraine attacks. It is also interesting that migraine attacks often become less frequent during pregnancy and during a period of rapid weight gain. In both these states blood sugar levels tend to be on the high side.

Migraine sufferers fairly often report that their attacks begin in the early hours of the morning. It is possible that this timing is associated with the gradual fall in blood sugar level overnight following the evening meal. It is simple enough for any migraine sufferer whose attacks frequently commence in the early hours of the morning to test this hypothesis by taking a sugary drink last thing at night. By the time the sufferer wakes with a headache, however, it may be too late to prevent the chain of events. Precautionary measures are worth trying so keep a glucose drink by the bedside.

In a similar way we can try to apply our knowledge about blood sugar levels in migraine to help individual sufferers. There are, of course, the obvious measures. Migraine sufferers who tend to develop a headache if they miss a meal should be extra careful about eating at regular intervals. If a journey has to be undertaken, or a shopping expedition, or anything that might interfere with a meal-time, arrangements should be made to carry a sugary drink or to take glucose sweets.

Young people sometimes develop headaches during or after active exercise such as running or playing football. We know that muscles use up some of their stores of glycogen during exercise. A drink, sweetened with glucose, before and during a period of exertion may prove helpful. The need for extra glucose, however, may not be the only factor concerned in the headache associated with exertion. The blood vessels of the migraine sufferer appear to be more sensitive to a number of stimuli than those of a non migraine sufferer and the jarring and jolting which accompany many activities may also play a part in the onset of headache.

8

Migraine and Hormones

AT the age of eleven there is little difference between the figures for the incidence of migraine in girls and boys. By the age of twenty-five, however, far more young women than young men suffer from migraine, probably four times as many women as men. This excess of women over men lasts throughout the child-bearing years of life and then falls off gradually from the time of the menopause until the seventies when the incidence in men and women becomes equal again.

Even this brief statement suggests that it is likely that one reason why women exceed men in having migraine is linked with the fact that in women changes in the body occur constantly in relation to the hormonal cycle. In the years when child-bearing is possible the changes governed by the hormones concerned with reproduction follow a rhythmic pattern. The average hormonal cycle lasts twenty-eight days.

During the first half of each monthly cycle the ovary prepares for the expulsion from its surface of an egg cell or ovum. This passes along the fallopian tube and into the cavity or body of the uterus. This expulsion of the egg or ovum usually occurs around the fourteenth day of the cycle. The lining wall of the uterus then thickens and becomes ready to form a soft bed for the fertilized ovum. This process takes about fourteen days, but if conception has not occurred then this lining is shed after fourteen days with the loss of blood occurring in menstruation. A new cycle then commences.

The menstrual cycle is controlled by a very delicate balance of hormones. Hormones are present in extremely minute amounts in the blood but they have very potent effects. Everyone for example has heard of the thyroid gland which secretes thyroid hormone. The chief endocrine gland in the body is the pituitary gland, which acts like the leader of an orchestra and influences all the other glands. Despite its major importance in the body it is only the size of a small pea. However it is very well protected from damage by being situated in a bony hollow in the centre of the skull. The pituitary gland produces a number of hormones and influences most of the functions of the body. Some of these hormones, like growth hormone, can act directly on body tissues. Others work by stimulating other endocrine glands into activity such as the thyroid, pancreas, adrenal, testes or ovaries. These other endocrine glands receive the messenger hormones from the pituitary gland and then pour out their own secretions in response.

During the first half of the menstrual cycle the ovary responds to a message sent by the pituitary gland by secreting the hormone oestradiol. This is the oestrogen which encourages the follicle containing the egg due to be expelled from the ovary to ripen, and midway through the cycle this expulsion of the egg, which is called ovulation, occurs. When ovulation takes place the ovary also starts to secrete another hormone progesterone. This helps the body of the womb to prepare itself to receive the egg cell which is about to be expelled. The body of the womb develops a thickened lining in which the egg cell can embed itself.

If the egg cell is not fertilized then the hormone progesterone gradually ceases to be secreted and after about two weeks it is no longer active. Forty-eight hours after the cessation of progesterone activity the lining membrane of the uterine cavity or womb begins to be shed in the process of menstruation. The hormone oestrogen is secreted throughout the whole period of the menstrual cycle, but the level of oestrogen also falls at the onset of menstruation.

THE WAY IN WHICH HORMONES CONTROL NORMAL 28 DAY MENSTRUAL CYCLE

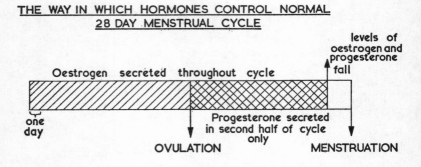

Fig. 5

There is thus a delicate balance between oestrogen and progesterone hormones during the monthly cycle. This is shown diagrammatically in Figure 5. If conception should occur then the secretion of progesterone continues and menstruation does not occur. The fertilized ovum embeds itself in the thickened wall of the womb and gradually develops into a fully formed infant.

Progesterone continues to be secreted throughout pregnancy and this is the reason why some women who have previously had repeated miscarriages are treated with injections of progesterone when they become pregnant again. Bleeding can occur when either oestrogen or progesterone are suddenly withdrawn. Bleeding due to withdrawal of progesterone and, or oestrogen, can occur naturally in the body as in the normal menstrual cycle, or an artificial withdrawal of these hormones can be produced by means of drugs.

If large doses of progesterone are given to a woman during the first half of the menstrual cycle ovulation does not occur If the administration of progesterone is continued as it pregnancy the normal menstrual flow will not occur either. The fact that alterations in the naturally occurring hormonal pattern can inhibit ovulation has led to the introduction of synthetic progesterones for use as oral contraceptives. They are given from the fifth to the twenty-fifth day of the cycle. This use of hormones in women with a normal hormonal cycle is inevitably an interference with the natural pattern of hormone function. In order to reduce the likelihood of bleeding during treatments and to maintain menstrual cycles of normal duration, these synthetic progesterones used as oral contraceptives are supplemented with small amounts of oestrogen. Thus oral contraceptives are pills which contain progesterone with varying amounts of oestrogen.

And what bearing does this have on our subject, migraine? The increased frequency with which migraine occurs in some women in relation to certain phases of the menstrual cycle is well known. In fact some investigators have put the figure for the incidence of migraine in women during their child bearing years at almost twenty per cent. Migraine attacks which are related to the menstrual cycle occur most commonly either during a menstrual period or in the few days following a period. Progesterone is normally secreted by the ovary from the time of ovulation in the middle of the four week cycle until forty-eight hours before the menstrual flow begins. So migrainous headaches appear to occur mainly at the time when progesterone is not secreted. For this reason treatment with progesterone has been prescribed for women whose headaches occur at this stage in the cycle. Further evidence that progesterone may be an important factor in headaches associated with menstruation is that approximately eighty per cent of migraine sufferers report

63

a spontaneous and complete recovery from migraine during a period of pregnancy. The hormone which is secreted throughout pregnancy is, again, progesterone.

A number of women seem to store water in their bodies at certain times in the monthly cycle, usually just before a period is due to begin. Their waist bands become tighter and their shoes are less comfortable. This water retention is sometimes mentioned by patients as a feature of their migraine attacks. Not infrequently a patient is aware that a migraine attack is about to draw to an end because he or she passes a lot of water. One of the hormones in the body which is concerned with the storage of water is aldosterone. Progesterone seems to have an effect in inhibiting the action both of oestrogen and aldosterone and this may be one of the reasons why it helps to alleviate some migraine attacks. It is interesting that oral progesterone is active against oestrogens but in order also to influence the action of aldosterone on water storage the progesterone has to be given intramuscularly.

The use of oral contraceptives in the form of the "pill" remains highly controversial. The naturally occurring hormonal cycle demonstrates an extremely delicately balanced mechanism in the body. It is hardly surprising that any interference with this balance results in undesirable side effects. The incidence of headaches in women on the pill is thought to be as high as forty per cent. The other side effects commonly encountered are mood changes, particularly depression, clotting in veins, irregularities in the menstrual cycle and a gain in weight.

An increasing number of young women are being referred to migraine clinics following either an increase in the severity of their headache symptoms or because they have developed migrainous headache as a new symptom since they started on the pill. The pill is given from the fifth to the twenty-fifth day of the menstrual cycle counting the onset of menstruation as the first day of the cycle. Headaches "on the pill" occur most commonly in the intervals between courses.

The headaches which can occur for the first time in women on the pill are often migrainous in nature. This means to say that they are often felt chiefly on one side of the head and are throbbing in character. They may be accompanied by eye signs, nausea and vomiting. The eye signs may consist of blurred vision or flashing lights or zigzag lines, the typical "fortification spectra" may occur. Sometimes the actual head pain is described as "vice-like."

A proportion of the women who complain of headaches when they are taking the pill, possibly about twenty-five per cent of the women who complain of headache, have symptoms which are less characteristic of the typical migraine pattern. Their headaches are felt all over the head and are described as being like a tight band or pressure on the head. They may be accompanied by a feeling of depression or irritability. Sleeplessness may be an associated symptom. These headaches also occur most frequently at the time of the menstrual period.

Very occasionally women who develop headaches on the pill also complain of symptoms associated with a disorder of the nervous system. Among symptoms of this nature that have been reported are loss of sight, usually in one half of the normal field of vision, weakness in an arm or leg or difficulty in speech. These symptoms may last from a few minutes to several hours and are usually temporary although in some rare cases the patient has been left with a permanent defect of vision, or loss of power in a limb. Obviously it is absolutely vital to stop the pill at once in any woman complaining of any symptoms which suggest any disorder of the nervous system. Many physicians and particularly those who work in migraine clinics would go further and consider that the use of the pill is ill advised in any woman who suffers from migraine.

Recent work has shown that the important factor in producing headache in patients taking the pill is the ratio between the amount of oestrogen and the amount of progesterone present in the pill. The pill that appears to carry the highest risk in producing unwanted side effects is the one with a high content of oestrogen. It has been recommended that only oral contraceptive pills containing less than fifty micrograms* of oestrogen should be used and this is now standard practice.

Opinions differ, but in my view it is unwise for a migraine sufferer to start taking the pill. Even women who do not suffer from headaches but who have a family history of migraine should embark on this course very warily. If a woman has nevertheless decided to take the pill the danger signals should

* One microgram is one ten thousandth of a gram.

be heeded carefully. If a patient on the pill starts getting head-aches, or if the headaches she already had before she started on the pill become more severe, she should consult her doctor at once. Similarly any symptoms which might be related to damage to the nervous system such as loss of vision, or weak-ness in a limb should be reported immediately. Even though these symptoms may only last for a few minutes and then re-cover completely, it is essential to seek medical advice. They should not be ignored under any circumstances.

Every now and then figures are produced for the incidence of headache among women taking the pill. These vary so widely that they are of very little use. The figures differ according to the type of pill being considered and the various criteria for headache adopted by the assessor. The important fact is not the actual figures, which are probably small in relation to the enormous number of women on the pill, but an awareness of its possible harmful effects.

9

Remarks on Research

"why don't 'they' do something about it?" is a comment that we have all heard many times and probably also made our-selves. But who are "they," and what reply can we expect? Of course, it all depends on the nature of "it." But let us confine ourselves to the "it" of migraine research and the "they" of the medical profession.

Well, why don't they do something about it? After all, if up to one in ten people suffer from a painful, recurring, disabling complaint it is not unreasonable to expect some action to be taken. Whenever it arises in general conversation the subject of medical research evokes immediate emotional reactions. Either "they" are not doing enough about "it," or "they" are always experimenting on you. It is not unusual to hear both criticisms levelled in almost the same breath. Interest is usually immediately focused on exciting areas of research such as heart transplant surgery. This interest soon abates, however. Fed as we are on a daily diet of death, violence and destruction we rapidly come to accept the most recent dramatic event whatever it may be. Within a short space of time we barely notice the small print in the paper which reports on the latest heart transplant survivor. But let us leave the emotional impact of medical research aside and consider the need for research.

Obviously it is necessary, you will say, because without it our knowledge of disorders will stand still. Considering the atom bomb and atmospheric pollution as two of our current end products of advancing knowledge one might be forgiven for wondering whether the pursuit of knowledge is not without its drawbacks. But the same curiosity which has driven men forward to make these advances has also led to the steam engine, wireless waves, vaccination against smallpox and the prevention of rickets. We cannot decide in advance the direction in which man's curiosity should lead him and can only hope that good sense and sound judgement will enable new discoveries to be rightly used.

The search for knowledge is essential in our universities and other centres of learning. The undertaking of research implies enquiry and a constant seeking for the answers to questions. Unless teachers and students are encouraged to adopt this approach to problems, learning will rapidly become routine and stagnation will occur. For this reason research is undertaken in most university departments and the importance of a quest for knowledge for its own sake is recognized.

A classic example of this thirst for knowledge was Gregor Johann Mendel. Born in Austria in 1822 he entered the Augustinian monastery in Brünn at the age of twenty-one and was ordained as a priest five years later. He was partly a self-taught scientist but also studied at the University of Vienna from 1851 to 1853. He failed to pass the examination for a teacher's licence but taught natural science in the technical high school for twelve years until in 1868 he was elected abbot of his monastery.

During the years when he was teaching at the technical school he was also carrying out patient meticulous research, crossing varieties of the garden pea in the monastery garden. He carefully noted the way in which differences in single characters such as tallness and shortness, seed shape and seed size were transmitted through succeeding generations of the pea plants. It is not difficult to imagine the endless patience and minute observation required to undertake this time consuming work. In 1856 Mendel published his experimental results and propounded the theory of inheritance which he had deduced from them. Acknowledgement of the major importance of his work which forms the basis of modern genetics, came only after his death. Mendel died in 1884 with his great scientific achievements unrecognized. Doubtless he found his earthly reward in the dedication of his labours to the glory of his Creator but his quiet perseverance and painstaking efforts remain an inspiration to us all.

Mendel may have had some inkling of the practical application of the results of his research to the future of mankind, but certainly he was given no encouragement to make him think that this might be so. He carried out his work because he needed to know. He thirsted for knowledge.

On the other hand, research may be undertaken because pressing problems demand a solution. To put it at its most dramatic, if an epidemic of a fatal disease is sweeping a country either means must be rapidly found of dealing with it effectively or the population will not survive. Necessity is indeed the mother of invention and research may well require invention on a scientific basis. During the last war one of the main problems facing the medical military staff in the Far East was scrub typhus. A solution to the problem had to be found. Desperate times demand desperate measures and the sacrosanct right of the scientist to choose his own field of endeavour was overruled. A group of research workers were gathered together in a country house and provided with the facilities they required in order to tackle the problem. A solution was swiftly found. Unfortunately this sort of success is far from being the usual case in applied research. We have only to consider all the work being carried out in an attempt to solve the problem of the common cold, or the problems of coronary heart disease and rheumatoid arthritis to realize that the will does not inevitably lead to the way.

Where does the financial support required for research come from? A large amount of research is government financed both in the universities and in research institutes. In this country the official bodies have tended to apply their funds to those areas in which the best scientific work was being done, without paying too much attention to the relevance of the work being undertaken to practical problems. This policy of applying funds for research has recently been called into question and the application of research projects to practical problems will receive greater attention in future. A number of charitable foundations and trusts also support research but their funds are often designated for particular purposes such as the furtherance of cancer research or research into rheumatism. A great deal of the money provided by charities supporting medical research is raised by public subscription. Certain diseases such as cancer or the crippling disorders of childhood arouse unfailing public sympathy and appeals for support always meet with at least some success.

In Britain the interests of migraine sufferers are fostered by their own Trust and the British Migraine Association. As the need has become more widely recognized similar bodies have been formed in other countries.

Research, however, is not only a matter of perceiving a problem or of seeking financial support to investigate it, or even both these things. It is also a matter of training suitable research workers. The methods employed for the investigation of disease become more complex every year and for most research workers a prolonged period of preliminary training is necessary before specific problems can be tackled.

There are a number of different ways in which research into any particular disorder can be undertaken. First of all we need to know how frequently a particular disorder occurs. Epidemiology is the study of the incidence of a disease and the factors related to its incidence. For example epidemiological studies pointed to the relationship between lung cancer and smoking. Some people may refuse to accept that this association has been proved, and may even go as far as blaming lung cancer on petrol fumes or pollution in general. There are always those who refuse to be convinced, probably because it suits them better to carry on smoking. Carefully controlled studies have shown that the incidence of lung cancer is significantly increased in smokers and that the heavy smoker is more likely than the light smoker to develop lung cancer. Epidemiological studies in other fields have often failed to produce such clear cut results.

We have all read newspaper articles telling us to use vegetable oils, instead of animal fat in our diets. The role of saturated fat in the diet of patients suffering from coronary heart disease has not yet been clearly established. Many investigations have been undertaken in attempts to settle the issue. Relating specific factors to the incidence of a particular disorder sounds relatively easy but is far from being the case in practice. In order to obtain accurate results great care and precision, time and patience are required as well as a completely scientific approach to the problem and an open mind. We readily believe what we wish to believe, but this understandable tendency must not in the smallest measure influence the research worker in epidemiology. Only unbiased facts are of value. Many studies of the incidence of migraine have been undertaken in Scandinavia and Britain, and they indicate clearly that the condition is familial in nature, and that the incidence is approximately the same in these countries. It would be interesting to obtain figures for the incidence of migraine in the Tropics but more pressing problems than this face the limited number of research workers in those climes.

Migraine is a disorder of blood vessels and a great deal of research into migraine has consisted of clinical studies to determine exactly what happens to the affected blood vessels during an attack. Attempts to carry out investigations into migraine are hampered in various ways. The first snag is that sufferers from a migraine attack are rarely admitted to hospital. If your patient is a captive in a hospital bed it is relatively easy to study the course of a disorder, but most migraine patients suffer quietly in their own homes and are out of reach of the physician who is trying to carry out research into the problems. The advent of an all day Migraine Clinic in the City of London, supported by the Migraine Trust, where sufferers can receive treatment during an attack, should go a long way towards solving this problem in at least one site!

A number of methods are available to enable studies to be undertaken of the changes occurring in the affected blood vessels during a migraine attack. Thermography is a technique by which changes in skin temperature can be recorded. When the blood flow is increased in an area, then the temperature of the skin covering it rises. The results of thermographic investigation indicate that an increased blood flow is present in the painful area of the head during an attack of migraine. In the section of this book describing what happens during an attack, a careful distinction is made between the blood flow inside the skull and the blood flow in the head outside the skull. Methods such as thermography provide a clue to what is happening in the blood vessels outside the skull.

The only place in the body where one can obtain a direct view of what is happening to blood vessels is in the eye. Using an ophthalmoscope it is possible to look into the eye and study the blood vessels running across the retina at the back of the eye. Retinal cameras are now available with which it is possible to take photographs of the retina and to obtain a visual record of the size of the blood vessels. These vessels are branches of the internal carotid artery and reflect changes in the intracerebral blood vessels. Research workers on this field have reported that during the prodromal phase of migraine, immediately before the onset of the headache, the small arteries of the retina become narrower. This narrowing affects not only the vessels in the eye on the side of the head that becomes painful, but the vessels on the retinas of both eyes.

Using a retinal camera is not the only method by which a visual assessment of blood vessel size in the skull can be made. Radiopaque materials (which are opaque to X-rays) can be injected into selected blood vessels and these vessels then show up on an X-ray picture. Serial films taken during a migraine attack confirm that the vessels inside the skull become narrowed just before the headache begins.

Another way in which the blood flow in an area can be estimated is by means of "labelled" substances. The substance used in the "label" is radioactive. If such a labelled substance is introduced into the bloodstream, either by inhalation through the lungs or by injection into a blood vessel, then the amount of labelled material in the area being investigated can be measured over a period of time with a Geiger counter. Calculations are then made to relate the measurements obtained by means of the Geiger counter to the blood flow through the area. Comparisons can then be made between the blood flow in various sites such as both sides of the head.

All the blood flow studies so far undertaken in migraine indicate that during the prodromal phase a constriction occurs in the vessels within the skull. During the painful period the vessels outside the skull in the affected area dilate.

A major field of research into migraine lies in biochemical investigation. The section of this book dealing with biochemistry outlines some of this work and it is also mentioned in other sections of this book, such as those on hunger and hormones.

Migraine is a complex disorder. It is therefore hardly surprising that not only the physician but also the biochemist, the psychologist, the physicist and the physiologist are among those who can contribute with advantage to research into this subject.

10

The Biochemistry of Migraine

THE alchemists of old searched not only for ways of turning baser metals into gold but also for an elixir of life. Their studies of nature were linked with astrology and mysticism and they sensed vaguely that a knowledge of the chemical transformation of matter might lead to power to benefit man. Their investigations were combined with the search for the philosopher's stone. This substance was supposed to possess wonderful properties that could turn lead into gold, cure disease, restore youth and prolong life. Methods have changed but the pursuits of the alchemists were not so far removed from those of many a modern man although we frequently wrap our philosopher's stone in a gaudier, commercial package. The alchemists tried to discover the substance of life and although this approach was necessarily largely philosophical they were nevertheless the forerunners of modern science. In the sixteenth century the iatrochemists taught that the main purpose of the study of matter was to make medicines and aid the physician.

An English philosopher Robert Boyle was one of the founders of modern chemistry. Boyle lived from 1627 to 1691. He questioned the basis of the chemical theory of his day and taught that the proper object of chemistry was to determine the composition of substances. His contemporary, John Mayow, observed the fundamental analogy between the process of animal respiration, whereby oxygen is taken into the body with the breakdown of carbohydrate and release of energy, and the burning of organic matter in air. Lavoisier, the father of modern chemistry, later showed quantitatively the similarity between chemical oxidation and the process of respiration.

Photosynthesis in plants was another biological process which attracted the attention of chemists in the late eighteenth century, and the combined work of Joseph Priestley, Jan Ingenhousz and Jean Senebier showed that this is essentially the reverse of respiration. In respiration oxygen is taken into the body and with the breakdown of carbohydrate energy is released and water and carbon dioxide are formed. In photosynthesis in plants the reverse process occurs. Water and carbon dioxide are taken into the plant and, in the presence of chlorophyll, carbohydrate is formed. The simple equations for the two processes are shown as follows :

Respiration

OXYGEN		GLUCOSE	WATER		CARBON DIOXIDE
$6O_2$	+	$C_6H_{12}O_6 \longrightarrow$	$6H_2O$	+	$6CO_2$ (plus release of energy)

73

Photosynthesis

CARBON DIOXIDE		WATER	GLUCOSE		OXYGEN
$6CO_2$	+	$6H_2O \longrightarrow$	$C_6H_{12}O_6$	+	$6O_2$
		(energy in form of light required)			

Despite these early observations on living matter progress in biochemistry was dependent on the development of structural organic chemistry which did not occur until the nineteenth century. Obviously the molecular composition of a substance had to be known before it could be synthesized.

Progress was impeded by the Vitalists who took the view that organic matter could not be synthesized. When Friedrich Woehler achieved the laboratory synthesis of urea the Vitalists countered this blow to their theory by taking refuge in the fact that urea is a breakdown product in the body, and not a product of synthesis. The ensuing success of organic chemists in synthesizing many organic compounds forced the Vitalists to retreat. It is axiomatic in modern biochemistry that the chemical laws which apply to inanimate materials are equally applicable to the living cell and can completely describe the living cell.

In the nineteenth century two men in particular were responsible for developing the application of chemical methods to living matter. Justus von Liebig, a German, was born in 1803 in Germany. At that time it was difficult to advance in chemistry in Germany, as, not unlike the position still existing in some European countries today, there was a dearth of laboratories for the practical training of students and the subject was taught largely from textbooks. Liebig went to study in Paris and then returned to Giessen where he founded the first great teaching and research laboratory applying chemical methods to living processes. Liebig studied the great chemical cycle in nature and pointed out that this cycle is maintained by a continuous process of animal decay and plant synthesis. The application of this work to agricultural science became clear and led to the use of fertilizers for the soil. It is interesting that Liebig was the first person to synthesize chloroform.

In France at the same time Louis Pasteur was founding the

science of bacteriology. Throughout his life he was extremely industrious and even on his death-bed he exhorted his pupils to work. Pasteur showed that living organisms are responsible for the processes of fermentation, putrefaction and disease. His name remains with us as a household word. The pasteurization of milk evolved from his demonstration of the fact that treatment of liquids with mild heat for a certain period of time destroys micro-organisms which might otherwise cause disease. Among the other results of his work were the introduction of a vaccine to be used against smallpox and the method of preventive innoculation against rabies. It was Pasteur's work in bacteriology which enabled Lister in Britain to introduce antiseptic techniques into the practice of surgery.

Among the other great scientists of that day was Claude Bernard. Trained as a physician he brought a new approach to the problems of disease and recognized the importance of applying chemistry to medicine. He discovered glycogen and the fact it is stored in the liver. Glycogen is the form in which glucose is stored in the body and it is mentioned again in the section of this book dealing with hunger.

Gradually the need to link chemistry with physiology became apparent and a new branch of science was recognized. The term biochemistry was introduced in 1900. As the ultimate goal of biochemistry is to achieve a complete understanding of the processes of life within the cell and at a molecular level, it is obvious that as far as one can see into the future every step forward in biochemical knowledge will lead to endless new avenues of interest demanding exploration. Every disorder of function in the body must result in biochemical changes which differ from the normal pattern. It is not unreasonable to suppose that even those disorders whose aetiology remains obscure at present, such as certain mental diseases, will eventually yield their secrets to the curiosity, probing and skill of the biochemist.

The view most often put forward in an attempt to explain the mysteries of migraine is that it is a disorder of amine metabolism. But we are going too fast! Let us begin at the beginning! In 1838 a Dutch biochemist named Mulder named a substance recently isolated from living tissue "protein." The word protein was derived from the Greek meaning "holding first

75

place." It was an appropriate name as proteins are essential to life. Proteins are formed from chains of amino-acids which link together into polypeptide chains. About twenty different amino-acids occur in nature, eight of which are essential constituents of the diet in so far as the human organism is unable to synthesize them itself. Each protein molecule is likely to contain all twenty amino-acids arranged in a variety of sequences. It is the sequence of different amino-acids which gives individual proteins their specific properties. Enzymes form a particularly important group of proteins as they are produced by living cells and act as catalysts in the chemical reactions upon which life depends. Each different enzyme in the body controls only one particular action, and thus the working of an individual cell depends on the kind of enzymes it contains.

Digestion is the process by which the molecules in the food we eat are broken down into smaller molecules which are then absorbed into the body and built up into the material that composes our own tissues. Our food consists of three major constituents, carbohydrate, protein and fat. The vitamins and minerals essential to health are also contained in a balanced diet. The body forms different enzymes for the purpose of breaking down the food we eat. There are starch splitting enzymes, fat splitting enzymes and protein splitting enzymes.

The body continually requires and uses up energy. It obtains this energy by combining the carbon and hydrogen of the food we eat with the oxygen we breathe. The main energy requirements of the body are obtained from the breakdown of glucose which is obtained from the digestion of carbohydrates in the diet. The way in which energy is produced from glucose by oxidation has already been shown in the equation on pages 73–74.

The oxygen required is taken in when we breathe. Under normal conditions a constant amount of glucose is kept available in the bloodstream for immediate use by the body cells. Glucose is also stored in the form of glycogen, chiefly in the liver and also in muscle. This reserve can be mobilized if necessary. If an excess of glucose remains available when the body stores are adequately filled then the liver cells convert surplus glucose into fat. The fat stores provide a further insurance against need and can be called upon if the glycogen stores should become depleted. This could arise, for example, during prolonged starvation. Fat, however, is a less efficient source of energy than glucose, and the breakdown of fat results in the production of certain substances called ketone bodies. These are poisonous to the body and produce a characteristic smell in the patient like pear drops. This smell is sometimes very noticeable in children who have been vomiting for a long time. It also occurs in people who have been starved and who are breaking down their body fat to provide energy. Similarly untreated diabetic patients become ketotic as, despite the fact that their blood may be loaded with sugar, they are unable to use it. Their bodies have to resort to the breakdown of fat to supply energy.

Proteins are only called upon to supply energy as a last resort. This means that the body has reached the stage of breaking down its own tissues in its attempt to survive. Protein is an essential constituent of the diet and eight amino-acids are vital to life. The body is unable to make these eight amino-acids which must therefore be taken in the diet in order that life can be maintained. The essential amino-acids are

Lysine	Valine
Leucine	Methionine
Isoleucine	Phenylalanine
Threonine	Tryptophan

The last on the list is the one we are interested in here. When tryptophan is metabolized in the body one of its end products is 5-hydroxytryptamine which is also known by the name of serotonin. This was first isolated from blood in 1948. It is contained in small coin shaped particles in the blood called platelets. Blood has 200,000 to 400,000 platelets per cubic millimetre. The chief function of the platelets is in connection with blood clotting. If there is a break in the wall of a blood vessel the platelets clump together to form a clot which plugs the breach and stops the bleeding.

A substance called ADP (adenosine diphosphate) is present in platelets and is responsible for their clotting powers. When bleeding occurs platelets adhere to the damaged site of the vessels. They release ADP which causes more platelets to collect at the site of injury. They also discharge 5-hydroxytryptamine

(5HT) which causes the blood vessels in the area to constrict and thereby reduces further bleeding.

It is possible to employ methods to compare the rate and degree of platelet aggregation in different samples of blood plasma. Plasma is blood from which all blood cells have been removed. If plasma is enriched with platelets and ADP is added to it then the rate at which the platelets aggregate or clump together can be measured. Similarly various substances can be added to such platelet enriched plasma in order to see whether and how they affect the rate of aggregation of the platelets. The aggregation of platelets is a subject of interest in migraine because it has been shown that, whether or not they have a headache when the blood sample is taken and whether or not they are on drug therapy, migraine sufferers show an increased ability to aggregate platelets. Furthermore during a migraine attack a so-called "releasing factor" is present in the plasma of a migraine subject which causes the platelets to release 5HT. The presence of this releasing factor has been demonstrated by experiments in which plasma obtained from migraine subjects during an attack has been shown to release 5HT from platelets obtained from the same subjects during a headache free period.

Levels of 5HT in the blood have been found to bear a definite relation to the onset of migraine in migraine sufferers. Although there is no difference between the 5HT levels of normal and migrainous subjects between attacks, it has been shown that in the prodromal phase of migraine, that is just prior to the onset of headache, 5HT levels in the blood sometimes rise to three times their normal levels. They fall again during the headache phase. Despite the fact that the level falls at the time when the headache is most severe, the level in the migraine sufferer may still be above the levels in normal control subjects at this time. When investigating changes in the levels of 5HT it is essential to compare levels in the same individual all the time and not to try to compare them in different individuals.

When substances undergo changes in the body their end products or metabolites are often excreted in the urine. The major metabolite of 5HT is 5-hydroxyindoleacetic acid (5HIAA). The amounts of this substance found in the urine are often increased in a migraine attack. Changes in amount may occur over a very limited period only and frequent collections of urine may be necessary over a period of twenty-four hours to make sure that any change in amount is detected.

5-hydroxytryptamine or serotonin has several actions. It constricts large arteries and veins and dilates smaller arteries or arterioles in the limbs of man. It also prevents the excretion of water from the body and stimulates the activity of the intestine. These last two effects are interesting as some migraine sufferers complain of water retention before an attack begins and the onset of migraine is occasionally accompanied by diarrhoea. Whether or not these symptoms are due to the rise in level of 5-hydroxytryptamine, or even associated with this at all is not yet clear. During a migraine attack the level of 5HT in the blood falls and if it is then given intravenously the symptoms of headache are often relieved. The headache is often also relieved when the sufferer vomits and it is interesting to note that vomiting causes 5HT levels to rise in the body. Possibly the relief of headache following vomiting is associated with this. The side effects of 5HT are restlessness, nausea, faintness and flushing.

5HT is only one amine which is linked with migraine. Other vasoactive amines, that is amines that affect blood vessels, such as noradrenaline and adrenaline are also implicated. In carrying out research into migraine various methods have been used in attempts to induce an attack. Reserpine is a drug that has sometimes been employed for this purpose. Reserpine acts by liberating vasoactive amines including 5HT from nerve endings. Amine stores appear to be particularly sensitive to releasing stimuli in migraine subjects. The ability of reserpine to release amines declines with increasing age in patients. Possibly this has something to do with the fact that the incidence of migraine also falls with increasing age. Significant rises in the urinary excretion of 5HIAA have been shown to occur after reserpine-induced migraine. The exact role of 5HT in migraine is not clear by any means, as yet, but it seems certain that changes in 5HT metabolism occur in association with a migraine attack. Indirect confirmatory evidence that 5HT plays an important role in migraine is provided by the fact that one of the most successful prophylactic therapies in migraine is the use of methysergide. This drug acts as a 5HT antagonist.

11

Amines, Enzymes
and Catecholamines

AMINES

The subject of amines seems to crop up every time we think about the various reasons why attacks of migraine occur. But before we go any further we must define what we mean by an amine.

An amine is a substance that can be obtained from ammonia. The formula for ammonia is NH_3 and an amine is formed when one or more of the hydrogen atoms in ammonia is replaced by other radicals. Because there are three hydrogen atoms in ammonia it is possible to obtain primary, secondary and tertiary amines depending on whether one, two or three hydrogen atoms have been replaced. Amines can also be formed by decarboxylation, which means the removal of carbon dioxide or CO_2 from a compound. When carbon dioxide is removed from an amino-acid an amine is formed. The general formula for this is as follows

$$R.CH.NH_2.COOH \longrightarrow R.CH_2\ NH_2$$

Amino Acid $\longrightarrow$ minus CO_2 $\longrightarrow$ Amine

Some amines are capable of affecting the size of blood vessels and can cause them either to constrict or to dilate. These amines are called vasoactive amines. Migraine is a disorder of blood vessels and a number of vasoactive amines are implicated in various ways in the causation of migraine. The chief of these are :

Adrenaline   Dopamine
Noradrenaline   Octopamine

Histamine   Beta-phenylethylamine
Tyramine   5-Hydroxytryptamine

Let us recapitulate briefly how these amines come to play a role in migraine attacks.

Noradrenaline and adrenaline are called the catecholamines and are discussed in a section of their own in this book.

Histamine is produced in increased amounts in the body in certain conditions such as shock and allergy. One type of headache which is thought to be a variant of migraine is called cluster headache. Cluster headache, as its name suggests, occurs in bouts or clusters. During a bout of cluster headaches the sufferer is very sensitive to histamine and even small doses can precipitate an attack of pain.

Tyramine is dealt with separately in another section of this book. Histamine, dopamine and octopamine are all found in certain foods which have been implicated among the dietary causes of migraine. Histamine is found in some cheeses and alcoholic drinks, octopamine in citrus fruits and dopamine in the broad bean. The latest arrival on the dietary migraine scene is beta-phenylethylamine. This is found in chocolate, cheese and some alcoholic drinks.

Possibly the reason why certain foods such as cheese and alcoholic drinks are high on the list of dietary precipitants of migraine attacks is because some of them contain a number of vasoactive amines which may exert a combined effect. Some cheeses for example contain considerable amounts of tyramine, histamine and beta-phenylethylamine. A similar position arises with a number of alcoholic drinks.

5-hydroxytryptamine is possibly the amine which has received the most attention in relation to migraine. It is present in cells in the blood called platelets. The blood level of 5-hydroxytryptamine is known to fall dramatically just before an attack of migraine begins. Furthermore, one of the most effective preventive treatments for migraine is a drug called methysergide. This acts as an antagonist of 5-hydroxytryptamine. The fact that 5-hydroxytryptamine plays an important role in migraine is undisputed and it is discussed in greater detail in the section on biochemistry.

Clearly a number of different amines are implicated in migraine. Not only do all these amines have an action on blood vessels but they are all broken down in the body by a group of enzymes called monoamine oxidase enzymes. So we will turn our attention to this enzyme group.

Enzymes are protein substances which are present in exceedingly small amounts in the body. Despite this fact they are of vital importance. Enzymes are substances which, without themselves undergoing any change, cause other substances to change. They act as catalysts in chemical reactions, that is they speed up reactions in the body. The absence or deficiency of a particular enzyme can have serious consequences. For example, when the enzyme phenylalaninase is deficient in a new born baby the level of the essential amino-acid phenylalanine gradually rises in the blood. This accumulation eventually causes brain damage and mental retardation in the growing child. The condition is called phenylketonuria and can be detected by a test made either on urine or preferably on a few drops of blood taken a day or two after a baby is born. On the very rare occasions when the enzyme is found to be deficient careful attention to the diet can do a great deal to prevent brain damage from occurring in the child. This is only one example of the way in which the lack of a single enzyme can have far reaching consequences.

When we think about migraine we are interested in a group of enzymes called the monoamine oxidase enzymes. They are concerned in the breakdown in the body of the vasoactive amines that have been mentioned repeatedly in our discussion of the causes of migraine. The monoamine oxidase enzymes add oxygen and remove ammonia from amines according to the general formula

$$RCH_2NH_2 + O_2 + H_2O \longrightarrow RCHO + NH_3 + H_2O_2$$

Ammonia is formed in this process and it is interesting to note that when a small group of migraine sufferers with classical migraine were investigated their blood levels of ammonia were found to be raised.

Monoamine oxidase enzymes are widespread in the body. Their concentration differs in various sites. For example, they are present in relatively large amounts in the liver, salivary glands, kidney and digestive tract. They are found in fairly large amounts in the adrenal glands, the uterus or womb, the pancreas, the lungs, spleen and brain. They are absent or present only in very low quantities in heart muscle, red blood cells and plasma.

The occurrence and distribution of monoamine oxidase in blood vessels has also been studied and the amount has been found to vary greatly in different sites. As far as it has been possible to tell, the migraine sufferer does not appear to suffer from a generalized deficiency of monoamine oxidase. This does not, however, exclude a localized deficiency in the blood vessels concerned in the migraine attack but methods have yet to be devised for estimating this.

The way in which the monoamine oxidase enzyme entered the migraine field is interesting.

In 1952 a new group of drugs was introduced into the treatment of tuberculosis. These drugs acted as inhibitors of monoamine oxidase enzymes in the body; and it was observed that some of the tuberculous patients who were treated in this way became noticeably more cheerful. Because of this rise in spirits the drug was tried in patients suffering from depression and a marked improvement in some of them was soon apparent. This led to the introduction of monoamine oxidase inhibitor drugs on a large scale for the treatment of depression.

Despite the fact that thousands of patients in the United States were treated with these drugs no adverse reactions to them were reported for three years. Then reports gradually filtered in of severe headaches associated with a rise in blood pressure which occurred in some of the patients on this therapy. Careful detective work established that these headaches were associated with the eating of certain foods, notably cheese. The substance contained in the cheese that was responsible for these reactions was found to be a substance called tyramine, a name derived from *tiri* the Greek word for cheese. Tyramine is a vasoactive monoamine.

It is normally broken down in the body by the action of monoamine oxidase and exerts an action on blood vessels both directly and through releasing noradrenaline from its stores.

Although cheese was the main food to be incriminated in

the headache reactions occurring in patients on monoamine oxidase inhibitor drugs certain other foods were also found to have similar harmful effects. These foods also were subsequently found to contain vasoactive amines. Owing to the inhibition of monoamine oxidase by the monoamine oxidase inhibitor therapy which the patients were receiving, the vasoactive amines in the various foods were not broken down and rendered harmless as they would normally have been and the headache reactions resulted.

Since that time any patients who are treated with monoamine oxidase inhibitor drugs are warned against eating certain foods. The list includes

Cheese	Chocolate
Marmite	Broad beans
Yoghurt	Alcoholic beverages
Pickled herring	

The role of monoamine oxidase enzymes in migraine has not yet been determined. It is possible that attacks are associated with a deficiency in part of this enzyme system. More research will be needed to see whether or not this is the case.

THE CATECHOLAMINES

Have you ever wondered why so many of our bodily functions appear to be related to the rising and the setting of the sun? An internal clock seems to be ticking away within us, regulating biological changes with a cycle of about twenty-four hours. These changes are related in some degree to the presence or absence of light, and are called circadian rhythms.

The ingenuity of man devises ever faster means of transport and communication but his naturally occurring circadian rhythm poses problems which may yet defeat his purpose. The fact that physical and mental competence decrease and that stress and fatigue increase during early morning hours may have far reaching implications. It is of relevance, for example, when individuals such as airline pilots are expected to perform their duties with equal efficiency over a twenty-four hour period of time. A great deal of research into the subject of stress has been undertaken particularly in Sweden. Medically defined, stress is the response which the body makes to a physical or mental challenge. In certain circumstances the changes which occur in the body as a result of the mechanism of stress can lead to disorders of function.

During a period of stress certain substances are released in the body. The amounts of these substances in the body can be measured and the figures obtained for their levels used as an indication of the degree of stress which the body has undergone. The chief ones are the catecholamines adrenaline and noradrenaline. These hormones have already been mentioned several times in another context. In the section of this book on the causes of migraine a brief outline is given of the autonomic nervous system This consists of two parts, the parasympathetic and the sympathetic. The autonomic nervous system controls the involuntary functions of the body which are not under conscious control. One of the main functions of the sympathetic nervous system is to control the size of blood vessels. The substance which is released at the terminal ends of sympathetic nerve fibres and through which the actions of the sympathetic nervous system are mediated is noradrenaline.

Noradrenaline is not liberated solely at the ends of sympathetic nerve fibres. Together with adrenaline it is also released from the suprarenal glands in response to various stimuli such as emotion or a low blood sugar level.

Let us consider the chief causes of migraine again. They are

Stress
Hunger
Fatigue
Hormonal changes
Dietary precipitants such as alcohol.

All these factors affect catecholamine metabolism and result in an increased release of catecholamines in the body.

Reserpine is a drug which is sometimes used experimentally to precipitate a migraine attack. It has a marked effect on catecholamine stores in the body. Tyramine is another substance which is present in certain foods and which can precipitate migraine attacks in selected sufferers. Tyramine acts both directly on blood vessels and also by releasing noradrenaline from its stores. Migraine-like headaches have also been induced in some people by nitroglycerine. This is the substance that is commonly used by people who suffer from chest pain when they exert themselves or make an effort. Patients in whom headaches have been precipitated by reserpine, tyramine or nitroglycerine have shown a significant increase in catecholamine breakdown products in the urine during the twenty-four hour period in which the attack occurred.

A great deal of evidence is available to indicate that changes in catecholamine metabolism occur in experimentally induced migraine. Whether or not they occur during spontaneous attacks remains debatable at present. Most of the investigations undertaken in an effort to find out about this have been carried out on collections of urine made by patients over a period of twenty-four hours. It has become increasingly evident that samples of urine must be collected at short, frequent intervals, during the twenty-four hour period in which the headache occurs in order that any changes in catecholamine metabolism can be detected. These changes probably occur over a brief period of time only in relation to the stage of the migraine attack.

The chief breakdown product of the catecholamines is vanil-mandelic acid (VMA). The excretion of VMA is normally affected by a number of factors such as the ingestion of alcohol and coffee, which tend to increase catecholamine metabolism.

Let us end this section as we began it by considering the circadian rhythm in man. It is interesting to speculate on whether the frequent onset of migraine in the early hours of the morning is associated with the pronounced fall in catecholamine output which occurs at this stage of the twenty-four hour cycle. Possibly changes in catecholamine output are associated with changes in vascular tone which in their turn appear to be closely associated with the onset of migraine attacks. Furthermore the fact that headaches so often occur at the weekend or at the beginning of a holiday, when there is a marked change in activity, suggests that this may also be related to a relative fall in catecholamine output after a period of stress or work.

The levels of catecholamines in the blood are affected by a large number of factors. This adds to the difficulty of interpreting the results obtained when estimations are made. Nevertheless, as far as their importance in migraine is concerned investigation not speculation is needed, and a great deal of work remains to be done.

GASTROINTESTINAL FACTORS

A number of migraine sufferers feel convinced that their headaches are closely linked with their digestion. Some migraine patients have also reported an alteration in the frequency of their attacks during a period when they have been taking antibiotic medicines. These observations lead one to consider whether there are factors operating in the alimentary tract that have an influence on the incidence of headaches.

It is highly likely that this is the case. The use of antibiotics affects the bacterial flora in the intestine. Whether we like it or not our intestines are teeming with living organisms which are largely concerned with the breakdown of food products passing through. When this passage of food is slowed, as in constipation, or altered by changes in the bacterial flora concerned in its breakdown, increased putrefaction or decarboxylation may occur. Once again we are back with our now familiar amines. They are formed in increased amounts when the process of digestion is slowed and vasoactive amines such as tyramine may be produced in increased amounts and be absorbed into the bloodstream. Toxic effects like headache may result from this.

Food substances like yoghurt have a high content of bacterial flora. If you eat a lot of yoghurt this could affect your intestinal content of organisms and the process of food breakdown.

Work in this field is relatively recent. A number of French research workers are concentrating on the gastrointestinal aspects of migraine. They consider that the occurrence of migraine in some sufferers is linked with abnormal functioning of the sphincter of Oddi. This sphincter lies near the junction of the bile duct and the pancreatic duct. Further results of their work in this area are awaited with interest. These French workers have already demonstrated that migraine sufferers who develop a headache within twenty-four hours of taking oral tyramine tend to have a slower rate of food passage through the intestine than patients who do not react to oral tyramine.

Another section of this book comments on the subject of

histamine and migraine. Certain cheeses and other foodstuffs which have a high content of protein-splitting bacteria also have a high content of histamine. The formation of histamine in the intestinal tract depends on the presence of histidine in the diet. The histidine content of food is roughly proportional to its protein content, as histidine is an amino-acid found in many proteins. The possible role of histidine and histamine in migraine related to dietary factors is considered further in the section of this book which discusses research into dietary migraine.

We have mentioned the headache which occurs with a delayed passage of food through the intestine. An excessively rapid passage of food may also precipitate headache. This can occur with the excessive use of laxatives and a fall in blood sugar might be one of the factors responsible for the headache.

12

Dietary Migraine

"Where shall I begin, please your Majesty?" he asked.
"Begin at the beginning," the King said, gravely, "and go on till you come to the end, then stop."

From *Alice in Wonderland*

LEWIS CARROLL, who was a sufferer from migraine, wrote these lines. Doubtless he would have appreciated the problem of writing about dietary migraine. The problem is where to begin.

We might go back in time to Stone Age man and wonder whether he had headaches that made him curl up in a corner of his cave and pull a bear skin over his eyes. It is highly likely that some Stone Age men were affected in this way for their daily diet consisted chiefly of well hung meat and was lavishly endowed with the ingredients that his migrainous descendants, many centuries later, link with some of their attacks.

While Stone Age man provides us with food for thought he makes the writings of John Fothergill, a mere two hundred years ago, seem very up to date. And indeed they are highly relevant to our present subject as we read in extracts from his classic description of the Sick Headache.

My opinion of this disease is, that, for the most part, it proceeds from inattention to diet, either in respect to kind or quantity, or both; and that whatever medicinal means are proposed for its removal, they will prove ineffectual, without enjoining an exact conformity to rule. . . .

There are some things which, in very small quantities, seldom fail to produce the sick headache in some constitutions. Such are a larger proportion than usual of melted butter, fat meats, and spices, especially common black pepper. Meat pies often contain all these things united, and are as fertile a cause of this complaint as any thing I know; so are rich baked puddings, and every thing of a similar nature. A little error in these things will seldom fail to be attended with much suffering, in many constitutions. Indeed, as the disorder comes on, mostly towards morning, the generality of patients are led to consider it as a thing impossible, that they should suffer so long after a meal; it is nevertheless true, and ought to be strictly inquired into, and the conduct of the sick regulated in this respect, or medicine is exhibited in vain. . . .

That strong liquors will produce similar distresses to those who are not accustomed to them, is but too well known, and has been too generally experienced. Most kinds of malt liquor, taken too liberally, seldom fail to have this effect in particular constitutions, perhaps from the quantity of hops; for most bitters seem rather to increase, than lessen the complaint. . . .

It is not, however, the kind of diet alone that will produce this disorder; repeated errors in quantity will produce the like effects. Bile, if very acid, will prove a stimulus sufficiently strong, in many cases, to excite this sick headache in a violent degree. . . .

To obtain pretty speedy relief will not be difficult. An emetic, or mild cathartic, an anodyne, soon, for the most part, restore them to their usual health; to undergo the same conflict in a few days, perhaps, or a month or two, just as the cause of the disease is accumulated; and in this manner I have known many persons spend a great part of their lives. Wearied, perhaps, with ineffectual endeavours, they, at length, give up all hopes of getting rid of their malady, and think patience must be their only cure. . . .

But whatever process the physician's judgement leads him to pursue, there is one object, that will deserve his attention, and will require the patient's. This disease is not the effect of any sudden accidental cause; it is the effect of reiterated errors in diet, or in conduct, which, by weakening the powers of digestion, and otherwise disordering the animal functions, have affected the secretions of those juices, and perhaps the organs themselves, in such a manner, as to require a steady perseverance in the use of such medicines, as experience has suggested are most likely to restore them to full health. . . .

It is not solely with a view to the cure of this sick headache, of which I have been treating, that I wish to offer some general reflections on the dietetic part of medicine, and to point out the necessary restrictions, in order to its cure; but likewise, as they may be of some importance in the management of many other chronic and anomalous diseases, as well as for the preservation of health in general. . . .

Early habits of self command are of the utmost benefit to all, and even those who, without feeling any immediate distress from the utmost repletion at present, would find it their interest to be moderate and discreet. . . .

The customs of countries, in respect to meals, are different. Breakfast, dinner, and supper have been, in this country, habitual. Suppers, at present, are discouraged among the affluent; and excessive ones, such as have been in use among our ancestors, very probably with good reason; yet there are some constitutions to which this practice may not be beneficial : two very moderate meals, at a suitable distance, may perhaps be digested with much more ease than one full meal, and be made more consistent with the duties of life in various situations. From observation, I am led to suspect, that when people assure us that they eat no suppers, that it would be better for them if they did, than to oppress nature with a cumbrous load, that may be much more detrimental. . . .

The general breakfast of people, from the highest to the lowest; is tea, coffee, or chocolate. I say general, because there are many exceptions, some of one reason, some for others, making choice of other substitutes, as their inclinations or opinions guide them. . . .

To the articles I have mentioned, bread of some kind, with more or less butter and sugar, are commonly joined to make up the meal. . . .

From many incontestible proofs, that butter in considerable quantities is injurious, it is less used in many families. It is found, by many, to be very difficult of digestion, especially when toasted before the fire, or fried, as well as in sauces. Many people, apparently robust, and whose organs of digestion are strong, often find themselves much disordered by large quantities of butter. Nothing more speedily and effectually gives the sick headache, and sometimes within a few hours. After breakfast, if much toast and butter has been used, it begins with a singular kind of glimmering in the sight; objects swiftly changing their apparent position, surrounded with luminous angles, like those of a fortification. Giddiness comes on, headache, and sickness. An emetic, and warm water, soon wash off the offending matter, and remove these disorders. These are circumstances that often happen to people who are inattentive to the quantity of butter they eat at breakfast, and which are very often attempted to be cured by very different remedies, and improper ones. A sudden giddiness, let it arise from what cause it may, and it arises oftener, I believe, from some disorder in the stomach, than from all other causes put together, is a sufficient motive to call the surgeon, who must have a large share of disinterestedness and skill, not be compelled to bleed the patient, sometimes under circumstances that do not admit of it with impunity. . . .

A moderate quantity of fresh butter, with bread exposed as little to the fire as possible, or not at all, but used cold, appears to me to be wholesome; it is capable of becoming, with the other aliments as soft and inoffensive as chyle, perhaps, as any part of diet. . . .

The same thing may, perhaps, be said of coffee and tea; the heat, the strength, and the quantity make it unwholesome or otherways. There are nations who almost live upon it, as others do on tea; amongst neither do we meet with diseases, that can justly be ascribed to these ingredients in the common course of living. . . .

Chocolate may seem to require more consideration. It is, as we all know, the fruit of a tree growing in the West Indies, ground into a paste, with other ingredients, and serves as repast to multitudes of people of all conditions. It has not been observed, I believe, that those who, in this manner, make chocolate a part of their food, are subject to any particular distempers. It may be considered, therefore, as a wholesome kind of breakfast to those who like it, and with whom it agrees. It is of an unctuous nature, therefore little or no butter should be used with it. Were it commonly made thinner than is the general practice, and a large proportion of milk added, it would seem to be much more proper for common use, than as it is generally served up at present. . . .

To all these, sugar is for the most part a necessary addition : and, perhaps, much depends on the quantity of this addition, whether they are to be styled wholesome or otherwise. Nothing is more common than to hear persons complaining of the heartburn after breakfast, ascribing it to the tea, or the other articles they have been drinking. The liquors themselves have no share, or very little, in producing this complaint. It arises from the bread, the butter, the sugar, in conjunction : and is a proof that more of some of these, or all of them together, have been taken than the stomach could digest : and this circumstance ought to be a standing monitor against excess in quantity, even of things deemed the most inoffensive. . . .

Coffee, perhaps, is an exception to what was said above, that the liquors themselves have little or no share in producing the heartburn. Coffee made sweet, seldom fails to produce it; and it would be right to use as little sugar with it as possible. . . .

The effects of improper conduct in respect to those things which now constitute our breakfasts, are of little consequence, compared with those which arise from the well-covered table at noon. The indulgences of breakfast supply but very few materials for destruction. The repeated excesses at dinner, are serious affairs. It has been thought that more people suffered by hard drinking; than immoderate eating. My observation leads me to take the opposite side. . . .

The Author of Nature has so formed us, and constructed the organs of digestion, that we can gradually accommodate ourselves to every species of aliment; live on rice, on vegetables, on animal food solely, or mixed with vegetables, without suffering injury. No kind of food hurts us; we are capable of being accustomed to every thing; but this is not the case in regard to quantity. Nature, by degrees, may be accustomed to subdue and change into nutriment almost every part of the creation that is produced; but to quantity she yields; if there is not sufficient, decay ensues; if too much is used, fatal oppression. . . .

It might seem not improper, in this place, to mention my opinion of the different kinds of liquors, respecting their comparative advantages; but this might likewise demand a volume. It must be left at last to the experience of the individual.

> The lesser quantity of fermented liquors we accustom ourselves to, the better. To abstain from spirits of every kind, however diluted, as much as may be. Where mild, well brewed beer agrees, to keep to it, as beverage. Where water does not disagree, to value the privilege, and continue it. In respect to wine, custom, for the most part will decide. The less the excess in quantity, the more consistent with health and long life. . . .

It is now two hundred years since the physician John Fothergill first drew attention to the importance of diet in relation to migraine. This subject has aroused considerable interest in the intervening period of time. During the past fifty years a large number of articles have been published in medical journals on dietary factors in migraine. The authors of these papers have implicated a number of foods as precipitants of migraine attacks but because the link between the eating of the foods and the resultant headaches was not understood the condition was thought to be allergic. The term allergy often provided a convenient umbrella under which various ill defined and poorly understood disorders could be sheltered. The fact that elimination diets in which the suspected foods were rigidly excluded so often proved successful in treatment strengthened this allergic view, which has been altered by the advent of new techniques and advances.

The foods which have most often been cited as migraine precipitants during the last half century are as follows :

Dairy Products   Nuts
Alcohol   Eggs
Cheese   Wheat
Fish   Chocolate
Beans

We have lined up our suspects. Now let us see how we can match them with the clues.

13

Tyramine and Other Dietary Factors

IF you have read the last two sections of this book on dietary migraine and monoamine oxidase enzymes you may have noticed an interesting connection between them. Probably the link struck you straight away, but if it failed to do so, you may want to look through these sections again. The fascinating fact is that the foods which produced the headache reactions in the patients on the monoamine oxidase inhibitor drugs are very much the same as the foods which some patients with migraine link with the onset of their attacks.

TYRAMINE

Fortunately the reason for the headache and high blood pressure reactions which occurred in patients on the monoamine oxidase inhibitors when they ate cheese was soon identified as the presence of the vasoactive amine tyramine in the cheese.

The next question was obvious. Would tyramine in any way affect migraine sufferers who linked some of their attacks with the eating of the same foods that caused headaches in patients on the monoamine oxidase inhibitor drugs? In particular, could tyramine taken in pure form by mouth precipitate a headache in this group of migraine sufferers?

As this is the area of research in which I have been working perhaps you will forgive me for writing about it in a personal way. To begin with I would like to say how grateful I shall always be to Dr. Marcia Wilkinson for letting me work in her Migraine Clinic when I first wanted to investigate this aspect of migraine, and to the Wellcome Trustees who have kindly supported this work.

Patients who were attending the migraine clinic at the Elizabeth Garrett Anderson Hospital were questioned about dietary factors in relation to their headaches. Those who gave a clearcut history of an association between certain articles of food and their headaches were carefully selected and asked whether they would be willing to take part in an investigation. They were told that capsules containing food extracts would be sent to them by post. As patients are unlikely to develop a migraine attack again within forty-eight hours of having a headache they were advised not to test any capsule less than forty-eight hours after an attack. They were also warned against testing a capsule when they thought a headache might be due. For instance if a patient usually had an attack of migraine every two weeks it would clearly be pointless testing a capsule twelve days after the last attack.

A helpful pharmacist prepared some capsules containing one hundred milligrams of tyramine. This is roughly the amount of tyramine that might be present in four ounces of a cheese rich in tyramine. The pharmacist also prepared identical looking capsules containing lactose. Lactose is a completely innocuous substance and is often used in investigations of this nature as it cannot possibly exert any effect of any sort. Before the tyramine capsules were sent some of them were sampled by various members of my family.

Early in December 1966 the first batch of capsules, together with detailed questionnaires to be completed twenty-four hours after the capsules were taken, were sent to the first group of patients. The plan was that as soon as the reply on the first capsule was returned the next capsule was despatched.

The first four results after lactose capsules were returned negative. Fortunately none of the first four patients who took part in the investigation developed a headache after lactose. Tyramine capsules were then sent to these four patients. The excitement was intense when the first reply to a tyramine capsule reported a severe attack of migraine within a few hours. As once I used to hang out of the window waiting with longing for the postman to bring letters concerned with affairs of the heart, so now I waited for post concerning affairs of the head. When my sons John and Peter came home from school their first question was "Any more tyramine results?" Both the patience of my colleagues at work and the kindness of my husband at home must have been stretched to the limit by this total concentration on tyramine and migraine. Fortunately none suffered for long. Within a few weeks it became clear that oral tyramine could precipitate an attack of migrane within

The results of a number of administrations of 100 mg of Tyramine and identical looking capsules containing Lactose in 50 patients with dietary migraine.

Substance	No effect	Migraine attack
Lactose	60	6
Tyramine	20	80

twenty-four hours in a significant proportion of migraine patients.

Two doctors who co-operated in this investigation suffered most from taking part. One general practitioner was ill for three days after taking the tyramine capsule but at least it explained why for many years he had suffered from severe, frequent recurrent headaches. By modifying his diet he has been able to achieve a marked improvement in health. Another doctor, this time a woman general practitioner in Devon, took a tyramine capsule on Christmas Eve with a resultant attack of migraine over the Christmas season.

The testing of tyramine to see whether or not it might precipitate an attack of migraine was only a beginning. Tyramine acts directly on blood vessels. It also releases noradrenaline, another vasoactive amine, from its stores in the body and noradrenaline also has a powerful action on blood vessels.

Tyramine is broken down in the body by two main methods. One route is through the action of the enzyme monoamine oxidase. The other way in which tyramine is metabolized in the body is by linkage with a sulphate radicle to form tyramine sulphate. In addition to these two disposal routes a certain amount of tyramine is excreted in a free form in urine.

You may be wondering what effect, if any, large doses of tyramine by mouth have on people who do not suffer from migraine. This was subsequently investigated in three hundred volunteers. Tyramine was found to have no effect whatever in people who never get a headache. In people who occasionally suffer from headaches it sometimes produced a headache which varied according to the usual headache pattern.

This sort of research depends entirely on the goodwill of patients with migraine who are willing to risk having an attack in order to help in attempts to find out how and why these attacks occur. Several patients have co-operated many times in this research and I think that all other migraine sufferers, as well as the research workers concerned, would wish to record a sincere expression of gratitude to these volunteers. In addition I would like to state how grateful I am to Mr. Peter Wilson, Secretary of the British Migraine Association, for all the help which he and his members have given me over the past few years. By inserting a detailed questionnaire into the British

Migraine Association News Sheet it was possible to assess the frequency with which migraine sufferers implicated various foods in connection with their headache attacks. The foods that five hundred dietary migraine sufferers cited as precipitants of their attacks in order of frequency are :

Chocolate	75%
Cheese and dairy products	48%
Citrus fruits	30%
Alcoholic drinks	25%
Fatty fried food	18%
Vegetables especially onions	18%
Tea and coffee	14%
Meat especially pork	14%
Sea food	10%

Although approximately one third of all migraine sufferers relate the incidence of some of their attacks to the eating of certain foods this does not mean that food is the only factor responsible for headaches in these patients. All the other possible causes of migraine may also be operating but in addition these sufferers have learned through experience to beware of eating certain foods.

There are of course other migraine sufferers, who are unaware that the eating of some foods may be related to some of their attacks. If doubt exists, it is worth noting what a migraine sufferer has eaten in twenty-four hours before an attack. To become a food faddist may be as great a burden to a migraine sufferer, not to mention his friends and family, as suffering from occasional headaches. But without going to any extremes every migraine sufferer should be aware of the foods which might possibly be involved. It is simple to have a trial period of say six weeks, and exclude chocolate, cheese and alcohol, which are the most common precipitants, from the diet. The effect of excluding citrus fruits and coffee may also occasionally be rewarding. A trial period may prove particularly helpful in the treatment of severe and frequent attacks where the sufferer may be totally unaware of the fact that daily drinks containing chocolate or cheese sandwiches are maintaining a cycle of headache.

So what can the ordinary migraine sufferer do in practice about the problem of dietary migraine?

1. It is simple to recollect whether one has eaten chocolate, cheese or alcohol in the twenty-four hours prior to an attack.

2. If this proves to be the case on more than one occasion then it is wise to eliminate the offending article of food from the diet for a trial period of six weeks, and to continue observing whether any other articles of food might be implicated.

Now let us consider particular foods and their possible headache precipitating constituents. Tyramine is found particularly in substances which have undergone bacterial decomposition such as game and certain cheeses. The amount of tyramine present is not constant to any particular cheese. The tyramine content of cheese ranges from approximately one hundred milligrams in four ounces of a cheddar cheese rich in tyramine to trace amounts or none in other cheeses. Even in one specific type of cheese the amount of tyramine present varies according to the maturation time of the cheese, the bacterial flora and details of manufacture. It is not related to the flavour or appearance of the cheese. The cheeses in which the highest content of tyramine have been found are Stilton, Cheddar and blue cheese. As the tyramine content of even the same brand of cheese varies greatly a susceptible person might eat a particular sort of cheese with impunity on several successive occasions before having any reaction to its tyramine content.

Tyramine, however, is by no means the only constituent of foods which can precipitate a headache. The next section of this book deals with the subject of chocolate which heads the list of migraine precipitating foods despite the fact that it contains little or no tyramine.

A substance which is used as a preservative in a number of frozen foods is also a cause of occasional headaches. This substance is sodium monoglutamate. It was identified as the cause of the so-called "Chinese restaurant syndrome" in which a burning sensation and feeling of pressure in the face and chest may occur together with a headache following a meal. Amounts as small as three grams of sodium monoglutamate have been known to precipitate this reaction.

Recently reports were received of patients who developed headaches after eating frankfurter sausages. The active constituent in the sausages which was found to be responsible for the headaches was sodium nitrite. This substance is also present in cured meat products such as bacon, salami and ham. Ten milligrams of sodium nitrite has been shown to provoke headaches in susceptible individuals.

HISTAMINE AND HISTIDINE

The possible role of histamine in migraine is more fully mentioned in the section on this subject. It is present in a number of foods, especially those that have a high content of protein splitting bacteria. Thus certain cheeses and alcoholic drinks are rich in histamine. White wines, for example, may contain up to ten milligrams of histamine per litre and in some red wines this figure rises to twenty milligrams per litre. Histamine can either be produced in the body and is found to be present in increased amounts in states such as shock and allergy, or it can be taken in with food. Its role in dietary migraine is by no means clear. Foods with a high histamine content are recognized as precipitants of migraine. However, when six sufferers from dietary migraine were given twenty-five milligrams of histamine by mouth it had no effect on any of them.

Histidine is the amino-acid from which histamine is derived. When six migraine sufferers were given a dose of histidine four of them developed headaches. Similarly a research worker in Sweden found that when he gave histidine to three non-migrainous people they developed headaches. Clearly the site of formation of histamine may be important. When histamine is taken as such by mouth it seems to have no effect. It seems likely that the effect of histamine differs when it is produced in the body. More research will need to be done on histamine in relation to migraine.

CHOCOLATE

Who can resist those delicious bars and tempting boxes? The caramels and the cherries, the fruit and the nuts and all those delectable creams waiting inside their chocolate coating. There can be little doubt that the people who believe that chocolate gives them a headache have succumbed sufficiently often to be sure of their facts.

As far as one can tell, roughly one in three migraine sufferers links the onset of some of his headaches with the eating of certain foods. When five hundred people who held this view were questioned, the substance which they blamed most often for causing migraine attacks was chocolate. Of course, this includes chocolate drinks, cakes, puddings and sauces. Because cheese is also mentioned frequently in this connection and, as we have already seen, it contains tyramine, it was at first thought that chocolate too might contain tyramine. But this did not prove to be the case.

An analysis of chocolate was therefore undertaken. The search was concentrated on the detection of amines. The reasons for this were the fact that tyramine had been shown to precipitate migraine and because other vasoactive amines such as 5-hydroxytryptamine and noradrenaline are known to play a role in migraine. Chocolate is extremely difficult to analyse and all credit must be given to the research workers at the British Food Manufacturers Research Association at Leatherhead who undertook the task.

Dozens of different amines were found to be present in chocolate. This investigation was carried out in parallel with an analysis of various cheeses and wines. Interest was immediately aroused when one particular amine was identified in all three substances. This was beta-phenylethylamine which falls into the same group of amines as tyramine. It has a direct action on blood vessels and also releases noradrenaline from its stores in the body.

As beta-phenylethylamine looked such a promising suspect, arrangements were made for a trial of this substance to see whether or not it could have an effect in precipitating migraine attacks. Once more the call for migraine volunteers was heard. A group of schoolgirls in Leicester who were carrying out an enterprising science project on dietary migraine kindly helped me with a list of volunteers. A total of fifty patients responded. All of them considered that some of their headaches were associated with the eating of certain foods and they all included chocolate among these foods.

Five of the volunteers had to be excluded from the investigation because they were being treated for depression or were taking the "pill." Both of these factors could influence the incidence of headaches and bias the results. The volunteers provided all the relevant information about themselves on detailed questionnaire sheets and they were also asked to obtain the consent of their own doctors before taking part in this test.

The amount of beta-phenylethylamine which is present in a two ounce bar of chocolate is about three milligrams. Once again capsules were prepared containing this amount and also identical looking capsules containing lactose. The lactose capsules were sent out first. Forty-five volunteers received them. Whenever a report on a lactose sample was returned the next capsule containing beta-phenylethylamine was despatched.

Thirty-nine people returned reports on both samples. Of these thirty-nine individuals two developed an attack of migraine after both samples. Four had an attack after lactose only and sixteen after beta-phenylethylamine only. The full results are given on the table on this page. They are strongly suggestive of the fact that beta-phenylethylamine is at least one substance present in chocolate that can act as a cause of migraine. It becomes even more interesting when we learn

Results of the administration of 3 mg of beta-phenylethylamine (which is present in 2 oz of some chocolate) and identical looking capsules containing lactose

Substance	No effect	Migraine attack
Lactose	33	6
Beta-phenyl-ethylamine	21	18

Two people included in this table suffered migraine attacks after taking both substances.

from the biochemists who found the beta-phenylethylamine that a similar amount of this substance is present in ten ounces of certain wines and some cheeses.

We have now lined up two suspects in our indicted foods, namely beta-phenylethylamine and tyramine. Any jury might reasonably be expected to decide that following a fair trial both have been proved guilty.

ALCOHOL

Since the days of the Old Testament when Noah first tilled the soil and planted a vineyard, men have celebrated their joys and drowned their sorrows with the aid of alcohol. The ancient Romans used to hold orgies of worship to Bacchus, the god of wine. Any migraine sufferers amongst them doubtless paid dearly with headaches for their excesses. The stern reprimand of Livy, the most famous of Roman historians who recorded these events could have provided little solace,

Men's minds are too ready to excuse guilt in themselves.

One or two out of every ten migraine sufferers abstain from alcohol because it gives them a headache. As far as migraine is concerned alcoholic drinks contain several substances that must be regarded with suspicion.

To start with they contain ethyl alcohol. This causes blood vessels on the surface of the body to dilate. The rosy flush which follows one or two glasses of wine as well as the red face of the chronic alcoholic are visible evidence of this. We have already seen that in people who suffer from migraine the blood vessels which are affected in an attack appear to react in a particularly sensitive way to any stimuli. The action of alcohol in dilating blood vessels could be such a stimulus. It is not only migraine sufferers who get a headache after alcohol. The difference is really one of degree. The typical hangover headache is due to vasodilation and usually occurs after a considerable amount of alcohol has been taken. Some migraine sufferers develop an attack after drinking relatively small amounts of alcohol.

When large amounts of alcohol are taken a fall in the level of blood sugar occurs. This, too, could act as a precipitating factor of headache and has already been discussed in the section of this book on headache and hunger. The drinking of alcohol also produces changes in the production of catecholamines in the body. We have a considerable amount of evidence to indicate that alterations in catecholamine metabolism are related to the occurrence of migraine.

What other substances contained in alcoholic drinks, apart from ethyl alcohol, might be considered as possible headache precipitants? Once again we meet some of our old friends—or should it be enemies—namely tyramine, histamine and beta-phenylethylamine. Not only are all three of these present in certain cheeses but they are also found together in many alcoholic beverages. The exact role of histamine in migraine has not yet been established. We know that small doses of histamine can precipitate cluster headache, which is a variant of migraine, when a sufferer is in a susceptible period. In practice, of course, this means that small amounts of alcoholic drinks can precipitate an attack. Histamine is present in relatively large quantities in certain drinks. White wines may contain up to ten milligrams per litre and in some red wines this figure rises to twenty milligrams per litre.

Our newest recruit to the field of migraine precipitants is beta-phenylethylamine which was tracked down in chocolate. Ten ounces of some wines was found to contain the same amount of beta-phenylethylamine as two ounces of chocolate. One has to bear in mind that in any particular alcoholic drink all of the headache precipitating substances that we have been considering may be present and acting together.

So what can you do about it if you are a migraine sufferer? To start with you need to make sure that it really was the alcohol which you had at the party that gave you a headache. This assumes, of course, that you were drinking in moderation. So many other headache precipitating factors might also have played a role.

Let us take a typical evening out. First we have the rush home from work in order to get changed or the scramble of putting the children to bed and making sure that the baby-sitter knows what to do. Then the squeeze into an evening dress that has grown too tight or the irritated hunt for the cuff links which your wife has undoubtedly mislaid. This is followed by the rush of getting there on time. The particular details of preparation for an evening out may vary but the end result is probably much the same in most households. Before reaching the food you often spend some time standing like an automaton, with a cocktail in your hand, eating the little cheesy snacks that are so hard to resist. When you arrive at the dinner table to enjoy the sparkling wine you are probably well on the way towards a thumping head. By the time that you get home again you are growing only too aware of its presence.

So be sensible. Look ahead in a very literal way.

14

Histamine and Migraine

MOST people have heard of antihistamine tablets as countless thousands of them are dispensed every year. The conditions for which they are most often prescribed are hay fever, rhinitis, urticaria and other allergic states. The name antihistamines suggests that these tablets are acting against a substance called histamine. Clearly if they are sometimes needed then histamine must be a substance which is capable of producing unwanted effects in the body. But what is histamine?

This question would have been easier to answer twenty years ago than it is today. In those days every medical student was taught that histamine is a substance that is released in injured tissue. When the injury was widespread, as in a patient with extensive burns, a massive release of histamine occurred. Histamine has a powerful action on blood vessels, particularly small blood vessels. It causes them to dilate and this dilation after injury caused a dramatic fall in blood pressure and a state of shock ensued. At the same time the blood vessels became more permeable and allowed fluid to exude through them into the damaged tissues. This resulted in a loss of blood volume which added to the fall in blood pressure already present and contributed still further to the shocked condition of the patient.

This was a simple explanation of the role of histamine and everyone knew, or thought they knew, how histamine acted. As so often happens, however, increasing knowledge has led not to further clarification of the position but to a multitude of further points requiring explanation. We now know that not only histamine but a number of other substances are released when tissues are injured. Some of these are substances, like bradykinin, which has been mentioned in connection with pain, and the catecholamines, which have been mentioned in the discussion on the causes of migraine. Histamine, too, is released after injury and all these factors affect the blood vessels and the permeability of capillaries. In short the role that used to be attributed primarily to histamine now has to be shared amongst a number of substances. So what do we now *think* we know about histamine?

Histamine is a vasoactive amine. This means to say that histamine has an effect on blood vessels. In this way histamine resembles other substances that have already been mentioned such as 5-hydroxytryptamine and the catecholamines.

A very simple experiment will demonstrate the action of histamine. If you take an ordinary sharp pin and scratch the skin of your forearm rather sharply with it, but not hard enough to draw blood, then a bright red line will appear on the scratched surface. After about thirty seconds this becomes surrounded by a flare or a flush. Thirdly a weal or a blister will develop. When a suitably concentrated solution of histamine is injected under the skin the same triple response occurs. This, coupled with the fact that histamine or a substance very like it is found at the site of injured tissue, is one of the reasons that led to the conclusion that histamine is the substance responsible for the reaction which occurs in tissues in response to injury.

Histamine is known to be released in the body during the allergic reaction. In allergy an individual becomes sensitized to one or more agents. On contact with these an allergic reaction occurs in such a person and histamine is released. The response may be either localized or generalized. It is localized in such states as hay fever where the lining of the nose becomes swollen and inflamed. Generalized histamine release may result in the constriction of the air passages and asthmatic symptoms. Skin rashes also occur.

All the reactions to histamine that have been mentioned so far occur under physiological conditions in the body. But what happens if a person is given a large dose of histamine by injection? The reaction following a histamine overdose consists of a rapid fall in blood pressure with a dilatation of the blood vessels. Because the vessels dilate in the skin and the flow of blood is increased the skin becomes warmer than usual. More unpleasant symptoms arise such as a severe headache, asthmatic symptoms, breathlessness, diarrhoea and vomiting. It now becomes obvious why we are considering histamine. It has an effect on blood vessels and it can cause headache. These are two very good reasons why we should consider its possible role in relation to migraine. The position, however, is not entirely speculative. There is one type of migraine headache which is known to be related to histamine, cluster headache. The pain of cluster headache is usually felt around one eye and may last from a few minutes to a few hours. The eye on the affected side of the head becomes reddened, puffy and watery and the nostril on that side often feels blocked. The interesting point is that during a susceptible phase, when a patient is suffering from recurring attacks of pain, a number of substances are capable of triggering off the painful symptoms. Chief among these substances is histamine. Among others are alcohol and nitroglycerine. Certain alcoholic drinks are known to contain considerable amounts of histamine and this may be one of the reasons why sufferers from cluster headache are susceptible to alcohol at certain times. Nitroglycerine, used in treating angina, is yet another substance which acts on blood vessels and causes them to dilate. It would seem that during a time when cluster headaches are recurring the blood vessels of these sufferers are susceptible to the action of substances which affect blood vessels, and that at such times these substances trigger of headache attacks.

The role of histamine in cluster headache is undisputed. But what of histamine in relation to ordinary migraine? If a person, even a person who does not usually get headaches, is given an intravenous injection of one tenth of a milligram of histamine acid phosphate, a generalized throbbing headache will result. If histamine is given in the same way to a migraine sufferer during an attack then the pain on the side of the head which is already painful becomes much worse. Instead of producing the generalized headache that occurs in normal people, histamine exaggerates the headache on the already painful area of the head in a migraine attack. The question why the pain in migraine affects one side of the head only is repeatedly asked. The answer remains obscure at present.

The blood flow during a migraine attack is increased to the affected side of the head. One might expect the face of a sufferer to be hot and flushed but, despite the fact that the skin temperature is raised, the sufferer from migraine frequently looks pale. It has been shown that small central channels run directly from small arteries to small veins by-passing the capillaries. These anastomotic vessels linking small arteries and veins are particularly sensitive to the effect of small amounts of histamine in concentrations of one part in one thousand, which produce extreme dilation of these vessels. It has been suggested that the migraine sufferer is pale because blood is shunted from the arterial to the venous system during an attack through these small dilated anastomotic channels.

Two types of metabolism occur in the body. These are termed exogenous and endogenous. Exogenous metabolism occurs when a substance is taken into the body such as glucose by mouth. Endogenous metabolism of glucose would occur when glycogen is broken down in the liver to form glucose. Both types of metabolism occur constantly in relation to various substances. The end products of both endogenous and exogenous metabolism may result in the excretion of substances in the urine. Histamine excretion has been found to be increased in some patients with migraine and in some patients with cluster headache. This is probably due to an altered form of endogenous metabolism. The main breakdown product of histamine in the urine is 1.4-methyl imidazole acetic acid. The amount of this substance in the urine has also been found to be increased in some migraine sufferers even between attacks.

Clearly the role of histamine in migraine cannot be ignored. And who would wish to ignore such a fascinating problem?

15

Allergy and Epilepsy

> I do not like you, Doctor Fell,
> The reason why I cannot tell
> But this alone I know full well,
> I do not like you, Doctor Fell.

JOHN FELL has become immortalized in these lines which were addressed to him while he was Dean of Christ Church in Oxford in the middle of the seventeenth century. A student about to be expelled from the University was pardoned by Fell when he gave an unprepared translation of a Latin epigram in this manner. In our present era of student discontent it is a matter for reflection that Fell restored the good order to the University which had given place to anarchy and a general disregard of authority.

And what possible connection, you may be wondering, could this have with migraine? Poor Dr. Fell was disliked for no obvious reason. In allergic states the body takes a dislike, and reacts, for no obvious reason to a substance to which it has become sensitive. Allergy is a word with which we are all familiar. We hear it almost every day in general conversation. Although the complexities of the mechanisms underlying allergy have only recently become better understood it is universally recognized as a condition in which contact with a particular substance causes unpleasant effects.

Rashes are probably the most common form of allergy that we encounter. In recent years detergents have been blamed for a number of these rashes. The rash affects only those areas of the skin which have been in contact with the offending agent. This is why the rash is called contact dermatitis. The rash due to detergents may affect both hands and the lower half of the forearms as these are the areas which are put into water. Very occasionally skin reactions of this kind are so serious that the sufferer is forced to change his job. For example a baker who reacts to flour or a chef who reacts to fish might find it impossible to continue in their occupations. Nurses, doctors and veterinary surgeons may develop a rash after contact with antiseptics which are essential to their practice and may have to change the type of work which they do in their professions.

An allergic reaction produces swelling, inflammation and destruction of tissue. We have all come across people who develop a highly irritating rash, looking rather like a large number of inflamed blisters, whenever they eat shell fish or strawberries. This is called urticaria. An allergic reaction may be localized to a small area of the body or it may be generalized. A bee sting provides an example of a localized allergic reaction. The bee injects a foreign protein into the skin and the surrounding area reacts by becoming red, hot and swollen. Serum sickness is an example of a generalized reaction. Serum is occasionally given to patients when they are innoculated against certain diseases. On rare occasions the body reacts to this serum. About a week after the serum is given a slight rise in temperature occurs, and swelling of the joints and a rash develop. Usually this all settles down within a few days.

The substance which causes the body to react in this characteristic way is called an allergen. Probably the allergen with which we are all most familiar is pollen. An allergic reaction to pollen is so common that some newspapers give a daily pollen count during the hay fever season. A count consists of the number of pollen grains from grasses per cubic metre of air, averaged over twenty-four hours. At fifty or more, hay fever sufferers are likely to have severe symptoms. A large number of people suffer from asthma and hay fever and in both of these disorders many sufferers are aware of substances which may trigger off their attacks. These are frequently inhalants such as pollen or house dust but certain foods have also been implicated.

The term allergy was used to cover a wide variety of medical conditions whose causes were poorly understood. Migraine has often been included among the allergic disorders and in the first half of this century a great deal of research was undertaken into this aspect of the disorder. Migraine resembles allergic states like asthma and hay fever because like them, it arises at intervals and in a paroxysmal way. The fact that a proportion of migraine sufferers link the incidence of their attacks with the eating of certain foods was one of the chief reasons why migraine was considered an allergic condition.

Advances in knowledge and techniques during recent years have helped us to understand more clearly what allergy means. With modern methods it is now possible to identify and measure specific substances in the blood which result from an allergic reaction. The study of these factors is called immunology and this is one of the most active and rapidly advancing fields in medicine. Transplant surgery has resulted in an enormous concentration of interest in immunology. When an organ, such as a kidney, is transplanted it can act as a foreign protein or allergen and the body of the recipient reacts to it and may even reject it. In order for a transplant to be successful the tissues of the donor and the recipient have to match extremely closely.

Some migraine sufferers associate some of their attacks of migraine with the eating of certain foods. In a similar way some individuals develop a rash after eating articles like strawberries or shellfish. This dietary factor linking migraine and allergic skin rashes was largely responsible for the way in which migraine was included in the past among the allergic disorders. Recent researches, however, point to the likelihood that the reason why certain foods precipitate migraine is not because they contain substances which act as allergens but because they contain chemically active constituents. These constituents have a pharmacological effect on the blood vessels concerned in a migraine attack.

Skin tests are sometimes used in order to see whether or not a sufferer from hay fever or asthma is sensitive to a particular substance. They have only very rarely been found to be of any help in assessing the causes of migraine. Skin tests are carried out in the following way. The skin of the smooth surface of the forearm is the site usually chosen for these tests. The area is cleaned very carefully with a substance that will not cause any skin reaction. Small breaks are then made in the skin surface without drawing any blood. One such area is left to act as a control with which the other areas can be compared. Into the other broken areas various agents are gently rubbed. These agents are substances like pollen or horse dander which are suspected of being concerned in producing some of the attacks of asthma or hay fever or whatever condition we are investigating. A chart is carefully made identifying the various skin areas and labelling them with the agents used. The whole site is then observed to see whether any changes occur which make any of the broken areas on which suspected agents have been applied look any different from the control area. If the person being tested is sensitive to any agent the appropriate area is likely to show a change within an hour or so. The area becomes slightly swollen and inflamed. The patient is asked to observe the skin site for a period of up to twenty-four hours and to report if any further changes occur. If any particular substance produces a reaction its role in the disorder being treated can then be investigated. It is difficult without introducing an allergic factor, to understand why some migraine sufferers associate some of their attacks with the inhalation of certain substances. The inhalants most commonly mentioned are tobacco smoke, paint, perfume and house dusts. Even the scent of roses has been blamed for the occurrence of headache. In 1565 the Italian anatomist Leonardo Botallo wrote in his *Commentarioli duo* :

> Now odors pleasant to physicians and agreeable to all men or to most can be used in moderation furthermore in patients themselves. For both heart and brain are made better by them, as well as the liver itself; for one of the five senses affects naturally the ordinary state of the body and the mind is soothed by pleasant odours, they drive away unpleasant things. But sometimes, although they are pleasant to many, it happens that they may be unpleasant to one. I know men in health, who directly after the odor of roses have a severe reaction from this, so that they have a headache, or it causes sneezing or induces such a troublesome itching in the nostrils that they cannot for a space of two days restrain themselves from rubbing them. I know women who also have such an aversion to the odor of a calf that if they preceive one close by they fall into a swoon or are provoked to vomit or have a heaviness of the head.

Undoubtedly swooning at the odour of a calf was always a very rare cause indeed of migraine. Nevertheless the author clearly made his point four hundred years ago in this extract. Sufferers from certain disorders, such as hay fever, appear to be sensitive to certain substances which precipitate unpleasant symptoms in them.

In our present state of knowledge about migraine it is difficult to make a dogmatic statement about the role of allergy. For this reason we should keep an open mind, and as with many other aspects of migraine, we should carefully collect and sift the evidence.

Possibly the substance histamine provides the link between allergy and migraine. Histamine is released in the body in an allergic reaction. It is also liberated in states of shock and when tissues are damaged in any way by trauma or burns. The release of histamine may be either localized or general. For example a bee sting causes a local release of histamine. Serum sickness, on the other hand, is accompanied by a general release of histamine.

Histamine can also be responsible for producing headaches.

We know that one variant of migraine, namely cluster headache, can be precipitated by histamine injection, and if it is given in this way to a migraine patient during an attack, it will increase the pain already present on one side of the head. It seems not unreasonable to suggest that if a migraine sufferer reacted to a particular inhalant or other substance as if it were an allergen, then an attack of migraine might result. There is no doubt about the major role that histamine plays in allergy and it is also a fact that it plays a part in some types of migraine headache. It provides us with yet another clue to the aetiology of migraine which is likely to be of considerable importance.

ABDOMINAL MIGRAINE

This is a rare variant of migraine in which the attacks of pain in the head are replaced by recurrent attacks of abdominal pain. This pain may be associated with nausea and vomiting and it is only its recurrence in the absence of any abnormal physical findings, in a patient with a family history of migraine, that eventually leads the physician to the correct diagnosis. Like migraine in childhood it is a diagnosis which can only be arrived at by a process of exclusion. Abdominal migraine is interesting in so far as the symptoms appear to respond more readily to anti-convulsant therapy, than to other drugs usually used in the treatment of migraine.

MIGRAINE AND EPILEPSY

This section on migraine and epilepsy will start with a few figures about the frequency with which these disorders occur. There appears to be a shadowy relationship between them but the way in which they might be linked, if indeed they are, is still very vague. Migraine is about ten times more common than epilepsy but epilepsy attracts more attention and sympathy because its manifestations can be so much more dramatic. Epilepsy occurs in about one in every two hundred members of the general population. It is thought to occur two to six times more often in people who suffer from migraine than in other people. The figures given for the incidence of migraine in the population vary between five and ten people in a hundred. Epilepsy, like migraine, sometimes runs in families and when they are asked about it a third of the sufferers from epilepsy state that other members of their families suffer or have suffered from epilepsy. Interestingly enough, migraine also seems to occur somewhat more frequently in the families of sufferers from epilepsy than in the rest of the population. One in four epileptics give a family history of migraine.

There are other points on which migraine and epilepsy share similarities. Both conditions are episodic and recur at intervals. In the intervening periods, which may vary from days to months, the sufferers may be completely fit. Patients who suffer from migraine sometimes have a warning that an attack is likely to occur. Disturbances of vision may occur and the sufferer may see zigzag lights called fortification spectra. On rarer occasions a migraine sufferer may complain of loss of feeling in a limb. Similar aura or premonitory signs can also occur before an attack of epilepsy. An epileptic fit is characterized by a brief loss of consciousness. On rare occasions migraine sufferers have been known to lose consciousness during an attack. Epilepsy and migraine can both occur in the same patient and it is not unreasonable to suggest that there is some common basis in the reasons for which they both occur.

The fact that electrical activity occurs in nerves was discovered by an Italian physiologist, Luigi Galvani. He was born at Bologna in 1737 and gained his reputation as an anatomist. While doing some experiments on frogs he noticed that twitching of the muscles occurred when simultaneous contact took place between the muscle and two different metals, iron and copper. Galvani then conducted an experiment in which he placed one metal on the muscle of the frog and a different metal on the nerve to the muscle. In this way an electric current was produced and the muscle twitched. Galvani enunciated his theory of animal electricity in 1791. He died in 1798.

Electrical activity is going on all the time in the nerve cells. The fact that the brain shows electrical activity was first demonstrated in 1875. At that time some experimental work was done on animals. By attaching electrodes to the surface of the brain, and using a very sensitive galvanometer, shifts of between three and five millivolts could be measured. A recording made directly from the brain surface is called an electrocorticogram. For very obvious reasons this sort of investigation cannot be done in ordinary circumstances but the technique of electroencephalography in man has evolved from it.

An electroencephalogram (EEG) is the record obtained when electrodes are placed on the scalp. Small silver discs are used as electrodes. This investigation has some similarity with the very common technique of electrocardiography (ECG), which is used to obtain tracings of the electrical activity of the heart. When an electrocardiogram is taken the record obtained from the patient who is being investigated is compared with a record typical of a normal heart. It is then possible to see in what respect and to what extent function of the heart differs in the patient when compared with a normal person. In both the techniques of electrocardiography and electroencephalography suitable jelly is placed between the electrodes and the skin to ensure good contact. Transistor amplifiers are employed to magnify the very small fifty microvolt waves obtained through the scalp from the surface of the brain when an electroencephalogram record is made. Whenever electrical tracings are taken from the body it is obviously essential to insulate the subject from any other electrical interference.

Four main types of waves are found on an electroencephalogram and tracings from various sites on the scalp are obtained when a record is taken. These are then compared with the typical tracings obtained from a normal person. The wave readings are classified under the letters of the Greek alphabet according to their frequencies.

Alpha waves	8–13 cycles/second
Beta waves	14–30 cycles/second
Delta waves	½–3 cycles/second
Theta waves	4–7 cycles/second

In a normal subject the waves consist of alpha waves when the eyes are closed. When the eyes are opened the alpha rhythm is replaced by small irregular oscillations.

The rhythm recorded in an individual can be modified by a number of factors. For example, when a patient is under an anaesthetic the alpha rhythm is replaced by the beta rhythm. During sleep large waves with a delta rhythm occur. If bright lights are shone on to a subject during an EEG recording or the patient is asked to take several deep breaths then changes in the tracing will occur. Rapid movements of the eyes often occur when a person is asleep and dreaming. The rapid eye movements (R.E.M.) can be picked up by the electrodes and this activity is superimposed on the electroencephalogram tracing.

In monkeys rapid eye movements have been found to occur in the deepest stage of sleep. Investigations on migraine sufferers have revealed that a high proportion of people who wake during the night with a headache have just passed through a period of rapid eye movement on the electroencephalogram. During an epileptic fit changes occur on an electroencephalogram as the seizure is associated with an abnormal discharge of electrical impulses from cells in certain areas of the brain.

An electroencephalogram (EEG) is painless, harmless, and relatively inexpensive. It is not, however, a short cut to reaching a diagnosis, as the tracings obtained very rarely point to the definite diagnosis of a condition. In epilepsy, for example, characteristic tracings may be obtained during a fit, but between fits the tracings may be completely normal. In people who suffer from migraine an EEG taken between headache attacks will show differences from the normal in about thirty per cent of migraine sufferers. During a migraine attack this figure rises to about fifty per cent. But here again they are not diagnostic. The cornerstone of diagnosis in both migraine and epilepsy is the account of the disorder which the patient gives to the doctor.

A doctor will probably be able to diagnose the fact that you have pneumonia or tonsillitis without much help from you, but in a condition like migraine or epilepsy there may be no signs or symptoms to show for the complaint when you visit him. Everything then depends on exactly what you tell him, and although he will still exclude any other causes of your symptoms by a careful physical examination, the history given is vital to the diagnosis.

The idea that there might be a link between migraine and epilepsy has been put forward several times over many years. Once the technique of electroencephalography became available it provided a fascinating method of seeing whether or not one could try and link the two conditions. A great deal of work has been done in taking EEG tracings from migraine sufferers. About four per cent of people who suffer from migraine show the same changes that are associated with epilepsy on their EEG. This does not imply that they really suffer from epilepsy or that they ever will. It does suggest, however, that there is some sort of link between the two. Deep breathing exaggerates the changes seen on an EEG tracing.

There is another very interesting link between migraine and epilepsy. Approximately one in three migraine sufferers notice that some of their attacks follow the eating of certain foods. The foods which are mentioned most frequently in relation to migraine attacks are chocolate, cheese and alcohol. As we have already seen cheese contains tyramine which has been shown to precipitate a headache in susceptible subjects. As yet no obvious dietary factors have been implicated in epilepsy but in view of the possible link between migraine and epilepsy studies have been undertaken to see whether or not oral tyramine might produce any changes in the electroencephalogram. These studies were undertaken by research workers at the London Hospital, Whitechapel.

In these studies the help of three groups of volunteers was recruited. One group suffered from migraine but had never noticed any connection between their attacks and anything they had to eat. The second group suffered from migraine but were convinced that when they ate certain foods, notably chocolate, cheese and alcohol, headache attacks became more frequent. The third group suffered from both migraine and epilepsy.

Preliminary EEG records were taken in all the patients in these three groups. These were used as a control or base with which further records could be compared. Capsules containing one hundred milligrams of tyramine were given to the patients in the three groups and four to seven hours later EEG records were again taken. These records were then looked at by an expert in EEG studies who had no knowledge whatever about the way in which the individual patients had been grouped and what they might have been given to eat. Thus his assessment could only be made on any EEG changes, if such were present, between the original control recordings and those obtained after the tyramine was taken. The findings were of great interest as the records showed significant changes in the EEGs taken after tyramine ingestion in the patients with migraine who linked some of their attacks with food factors and in the patients who suffered from both migraine and epilepsy. More work is being done to investigate these fascinating results further. They imply two things, namely that dietary factors may have some link with epilepsy as well as migraine and they tend to confirm the view that there may also be some sort of link between migraine and epilepsy.

This type of research is dependent upon the goodwill of volunteers who are prepared to risk getting a headache and to take the time involved in co-operating with these studies. It is surprising how many people are prepared to make this effort, and it is through them that we are able to advance our knowledge, albeit by slow degrees. However, research workers as well as the willing volunteers who are so essential to clinical research can encourage themselves with the thought that progress is being made.

16

Some Other Factors

We all knock our heads at some time or another. The small child bumps it on the corner of the table. The housewife hits it on the shelf she has forgotten when she stoops to do her housework. The young boy is kicked on the sports ground at school. Even without including the more severe injuries which are becoming increasingly frequent as the result of road accidents especially in the young, the list could go on indefinitely. The point we are really interested in is whether or not these knocks or bumps could be related to the occurrence of migraine.

It seems fairly obvious from what has already been said that if all the head injuries in life resulted in migraine then the whole population would be suffering from it by now. So clearly this cannot be the case. But as with everything else in life, if you expect trouble you usually find it, and there appears to be a considerable psychological factor in the recurring headaches which start after a head injury. This does not mean that genuine headaches do not occur as this would be grossly unfair to the victims of head injuries who are lying in bed or sitting around with painful heads.

Headaches after head injuries are more common in people who have a family history of migraine. This is not surprising as migraine in any case occurs significantly more frequently in people with a family history of migraine. Since migraine is a disorder of blood vessels, investigators have been interested in the possibility of changes in blood vessels occurring after head injuries.

Investigations have shown that after a severe head injury the blood vessels in the affected area may constrict. However, this spasm is only temporary so it does not look as if we can blame any attacks of migraine which occur after injury on any changes in the blood vessels resulting from the injury. Headaches may occur after concussion but these diminish with time. Concussion is a temporary, usually very brief, loss of consciousness which may occur immediately after a blow on the head.

Three different types of headache have been found to occur in different individuals after a head injury. These are probably related to the part of the head that was damaged. When an artery has been involved short bursts of localized headache may occur. These may last for a short period, possibly only a few minutes of intense throbbing pain in the affected area. When a vein is damaged in the injury, pain may follow physical strain or exertion such as lifting a heavy suitcase. When a nerve has been affected painful spells may occur in a sharply defined area where the nerve carrying pain fibres is pinched in the soft tissue.

All these headaches may occur in different people for a period of three to six months after an injury. After this time they usually disappear. Very occasionally the onset of migraine headaches dates from the time of a head injury. If an electro-encephalogram tracing is taken in these patients it shows abnormalities in about twice as many of them as in people who suffer from migraine but who have never had a head injury. The electroencephalogram abnormalities may show up particularly around the area of scar tissue.

Another point is that damage to the neck is common in head injuries. This may result in the injured person holding his head in an abnormal position with resultant strain on the neck muscles. This strain in the muscles can also result in pain in the back of the head and neck.

If headaches occur after a head injury the sufferer should console himself with the knowledge that these headaches invariably diminish with the passage of time and pass off altogether.

THE KIDNEY AND MIGRAINE

Transplant surgery has provided some of the most dramatic advances in modern medicine. While the subject of heart transplants remains an open issue kidney transplants have become an acceptable method for the treatment of certain kidney diseases. The fact that kidney transplants are not undertaken more frequently than they are at present is due not to a lack of patients but to a lack of donor kidneys. Why are our kidneys so vital to life and what function do they perform?

A living cell is in a constant state of activity. In order to maintain this activity, in fact in order to maintain life, a ceaseless turnover of essential materials occurs in the cells. These materials are carried to them in the bloodstream. Waste products are inevitably formed in the cells and these need to be eliminated from the body. They are carried by the blood to the kidneys, which act primarily as a filtering system.

The functional unit of the kidney is the nephron, of which each human kidney contains about one million. A diagram of a nephron is shown in Figure 6. Each nephron is formed from two parts. There is a coiled globular shaped part called a glomerulus and a long tubule which is arranged in loop formation. Blood consists of a liquid portion or plasma, in which are suspended the different cells, red cells, white cells and platelets. Dissolved in the blood are various salts, organic substances, hormones, vitamins, the products of repair and breakdown in the body, antibodies and enzymes. The function of the kidney is to regulate normal concentrations of the constituents of the blood, by the excretion of water, the soluble end products of nitrogen metabolism and the electrolytes necessary to maintain the electrolyte balance of the blood.

The glomeruli of the kidney work extremely hard. Each glomerulus consists of a tuft of minute capillary channels supplied individually by the terminal branches of the renal artery which brings blood to the kidney. The glomerulus is enclosed in a capsule. In a period of twenty-four hours the glomeruli filter approximately 170 to 200 litres of protein free fluid from the blood. This means that they filter about fifty to sixty times the volume of plasma in the blood.

As the amount of urine that we pass on average during the day is one and a half litres it is obvious that extensive reabsorption of the fluid filtered by the glomeruli occurs. This reabsorption takes place in the tubules. They return to the bloodstream those substances which the body needs while waste products are left to pass out into the urine. The end-product of protein metabolism in the body is urea. This is formed in the

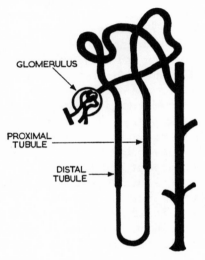

DIAGRAM OF A NEPHRON

GLOMERULUS

PROXIMAL
TUBULE

DISTAL
TUBULE

Fig. 6

liver and about two thirds of the urea produced in the body is excreted through the kidneys. The concentration of urea in the blood is normally between twenty to forty milligrams per hundred millilitres. The average daily excretion of urea is from twenty-five to thirty-five grammes.

Not only do the kidneys deal with the waste products of metabolism in the body but they maintain the pH or hydrogen ion concentration of the blood at a constant level. The blood is very slightly alkaline with a pH of 7.4.

If the kidney fails to function efficiently certain substances accumulate in the blood, chiefly urea. Urea is the end-product of the breakdown of protein which goes on constantly in the living cell. Very often a failure of kidney function is temporary and can be treated by extremely careful dietary measures which consist chiefly in the restriction of protein intake. If the kidney failure persists, however, the body gradually becomes poisoned by the accumulation of its own breakdown products.

There are two ways of dealing with this failure of kidney function when it poses a long-term problem. Renal transplant surgery provides one method of replacing a kidney which can no longer function adequately by a healthy kidney from a suitable donor. The emphasis is on the word suitable, as very careful matching of the recipient and donor tissues is essential. The method more commonly used to treat a failure of kidney function is renal dialysis. The body of the patient is connected to a machine which acts like an artificial kidney and filters the waste products out of the blood by passing it through various semipermeable layers. This restores the blood of the patient to a normal healthy state. The process of renal dialysis using an artificial kidney machine usually takes several hours. It is frequently carried out overnight. In this way sufferers from severe kidney disease can be kept well and at work. The chief problem, at present, is the lack of adequate numbers of kidney machines.

The reason why the subject of renal dialysis is included in a book on migraine is that about two thirds of the patients who undergo treatment with an artificial kidney machine develop a headache during the procedure. This may be migrainous in character and usually occurs one to nine hours after the start of treatment. The peak incidence is between four and seven hours.

The symptom of headache has been reported only in patients who still retain their diseased kidney or kidneys. If the diseased kidneys are removed and their function taken over by an artificial kidney machine then the headaches do not seem to occur. Kidney disease is sometimes associated with a raised blood pressure. Possibly the patient's blood pressure rises a little just before a treatment on the artificial kidney machine is due as the headache appears to be linked with the fall in blood pressure which may accompany treatment.

Treatment with an artificial kidney machine has given a new lease of life to many sufferers from kidney disease, and headache may seem a relatively small price to pay for the benefits obtained. Nevertheless anyone who has ever had a severe headache will feel acute sympathy with the sufferers on renal dialysis. However, because the changes in their blood are very closely monitored during treatment with an artificial kidney machine it may prove possible to pinpoint the factors associated with the occurrence of headache. This knowledge could eventually lead to adequate preventive measures during renal dialysis. It could also prove of eventual benefit to vast numbers of migraine sufferers.

MIGRAINE AND TEETH

It was Mark Twain who commented that Adam and Eve had many advantages but the principal one was that they escaped teething! Our teeth are a source of trouble to many of us not only in the cradle but to the grave, if they last that long. There can be very few who do not know what toothache feels like. And it is not only our teeth that can cause trouble. Occasionally the jaw too, can give rise to pain. This has sometimes been confused with migraine and must be carefully differentiated from it.

We have all been told at one time or another to grit our teeth and get on with it! This advice implies several things. First of all it suggests that we are facing an unwelcome situation. We are anxious about it and need to make a determined effort to overcome it. It also implies that when we are anxious we often make a physical as well as a mental effort to cope with a problem. We associate tension in our muscles with mental tension. If you are sitting in a chair waiting for an important interview you are unlikely to lean back in an easy relaxed manner. You are more likely to be perched alert and upright at the edge of the chair with every muscle taut. Next time you are trying to get somewhere on time and find yourself in a stationary traffic jam, take stock of yourself. You will soon become aware of the way in which the muscles of your body have tightened up, particularly in your head and hands. In some patients, especially those who are depressed or worried, this tension may affect the muscles of the jaw so much that it occasionally results in pain. This is similar to the way in which tension in the muscles of the back of the head and neck can result in tension headache. Tooth grinding is another symptom which can be associated with tension and may result in pain.

The best way in which to relieve pain in the jaw caused by tension is by coping with the problem causing the tension. Many of these patients, however, are chronic worriers who might do well to reflect on Emerson's translation of an old French proverb:

> Some of your griefs you have cured,
> And the sharpest you still have survived,
> But what torments of pain you endured
> From evils that never arrived.

As a leopard finds it difficult to change his spots the chronic worrier may find it difficult to change his outlook on life and a period of mild sedative treatment or treatment producing muscle relaxation may be needed.

Anxiety and tension, however, are not essential features of pain in the jaw. Some patients have a faulty bite. When they close their jaws the upper and lower jaw joint are out of alignment when the teeth are clenched. Clicking of the jaw may be an indication of this. The upper teeth may also slide on the lower teeth when the jaw is closed. Occasionally faulty alignment of the jaw joint occurs after one or more of the molar teeth at the back of the mouth are extracted. The upper and lower jaws are affected by the gap and no longer meet smoothly. This trouble can be dealt with by a dental surgeon.

Patients with trouble of this nature usually complain of pain on one side of the head in or near the ear. The muscle over the jaw joint may be painful to pressure. Clicking of the jaw joint may occur and its movement is less full than it ought to be. Treatment of all these symptoms is possible once the condition is recognized.

17

Drug Therapy

"As to diseases, make a habit of two things to help, or, at least to do no harm."

HIPPOCRATES

IN primitive times men regarded disease as the result of evil influences and did not realize that they arose from natural causes. The most primitive men alive today are probably the aboriginals of Central Australia and they still believe that the influence of evil spirits causes disease. When he treats a sick person the Australian aboriginal medicine man applies suction to the patient in order to extract the evil spirit held responsible for his symptoms. The medicine man then coughs into his hand and produces a small rock crystal. This is in order to convince his patient that the cause of the trouble has been removed. Other primitive people believed that disease is caused by a separation of the soul from the body. Instead of the medicine man, a soul catcher was called to deal with the sufferer. This custom still prevails in Borneo today. The soul catcher goes into a trance next to his patient and sends his own soul to find the soul of the sick man which has wandered away. When he has caught the soul, he emerges from his trance and exhibits a pebble or bead purported to contain the erring soul.

This primitive psychotherapy may make us smile but it is certainly preferable to the more violent methods of treatment which were once used and which have now passed into history. Trephination of the skull, in which a hole was cut into the cranium or brain case, was such a treatment and appears to have been fairly common in Bronze and Iron Age cultures. The first trephined skull was found in France in 1865 and soon afterwards more of these skulls were found in Brittany and other parts of France. Many trephined skulls have since been unearthed in

Europe, Asia, Africa and the Americas. Examples from the Bronze and Iron Age in Europe are rare, partly because the dead of that time were cremated.

The operation of trephining is known to have continued into classical times, and until only a few years ago the Arab surgeons of Algeria still practised trephining for the treatment of injuries resulting from a blow on the head. The operation used to be carried out on men, women and children, on the living and on the dead. Many patients survived the assault and some had multiple trephinations.

The purpose of trephination remains obscure and it has been suggested that it was performed for three reasons. On the living it was sometimes performed as part of a magic or religious ceremony. At other times it may have been used as a therapeutic treatment for head injuries and for diseases thought to be due to demonaic possession such as chronic headaches or epilepsy. Surprisingly enough the procedure rarely resulted in fractures of the skull. Trephining of the dead was performed to obtain bone rondelles which were pierced and worn as amulets.

Trephination was not only hazardous to the patient but also on occasion to the doctor. Chinese tradition describes the death of a Court physician who was called to see a prince suffering from unbearable headaches. As the physician was about to open his skull the prince was seized with suspicion. He thought that he was about to be murdered and one may well sympathize with his feelings. At all events, he ordered his doctor to be thrown into prison and executed. This physician is unique in Chinese medical history as the practice of medicine in China was violently opposed to any surgical interference with the human body. This is thought to be the only recorded account of an attempt at surgery in ancient China.

Until the time of Hippocrates the art of healing was a branch of magic or religion. Prior to Hippocrates, the Greek Aesculapius dominated the scene. Later worshipped as the god of healing he is a shadowy semi-mythical figure who may have existed in approximately 1250 B.C. Legend tells us that he had great healing powers and even restored the dead to life. Because of this Pluto, the king of the underworld, became resentful as he felt that he was losing too many new recruits to his kingdom and he appealed to Zeus to intervene. Zeus responded by slaying

Aesculapius with a thunderbolt. From the time of his death Aesculapius was worshipped as a god and temples to him were erected all over Greece, notably in Athens, Pergamos and Epidaurus. There was also a temple to Aesculapius at Cos.

Sick people came to these temples to be healed by the ritual of incubation. When the sick person arrived at the temple he first offered a sacrifice to the god. He purified himself by bathing, and then lay down to sleep in the abaton or long colonnade. This stretched along the side of the temple and was open to the air. During the night the god Aesculapius was supposed to appear to the supplicant in a dream and to give advice and treatment. In the morning those patients who had benefited from their visit left the temple. Others remained sometimes for long periods of time. We are told that while the sick were sleeping in the temples of Aesculapius their eyes or sores were licked by the harmless snakes that were common in Greece. The snakes were believed to assist in the process of healing, and the serpent is still a symbol of healing today. It is incorporated in the insignia of many military and non-military medical organizations in the world.

We know about the ritual of healing or incubation in the temples of Aesculapius because of the inscriptions on stone tablets found at Epidaurus. This was the site of the god's most famous shrine. One tablet records the story of a patient who suffered from insomnia due to headache. His name was Agestratos and he came to the temple, slept in the colonnade and dreamt. The god not only cured him of his headache but made him stand up and taught him how to wrestle. He departed in the morning, cured, and soon after became the wrestling champion in the Nemean games.

Legend has it that Aesculapius had two daughters with the rather mundane names of Hygieia (the Greek word for health) and Panacea (meaning cure). Hippocrates, the father of medicine is reputed to be a descendant of one of these daughters. Hippocrates was born in 460 B.C. on the island of Cos, close to the coast of Asia Minor. A living relic supposedly of his time is the huge oriental plane tree which stands in the centre of Cos. It was under these branches, now supported from every angle, that Hippocrates is reputed to have lectured to his students in the open air. Seeds from the plane tree of Cos are still distributed to various centres of healing and in the garden of the Royal

College of Physicians in London grow two plane trees which, strange to say, look curiously dissimilar. Both are thought to originate from seeds of the Hippocratic tree.

How fortunate the students of Hippocrates were. Despite the fact that he knew little anatomy or physiology, and had none of the tools of medicine we rely on today, such as a thermometer or a stethoscope, he taught with sound common sense. He made little use of the drugs of that time and relied upon nature as the greatest healer. He considered that climate played a major role in influencing the mind and the body and he refuted the idea that disease was a punishment inflicted by the gods. Hippocrates believed that "Every disease has its own nature and arises from external causes, from cold, from the sun, or from changing winds." He introduced method into medicine and it is the oath of Hippocrates which has been sworn by generations of medical students when they obtain their final qualification. This oath laid down clear guide lines for the highest standards of medical practice and one might reflect with sorrow on the way in which part of it is being abused today in relation to the sanctity of human life.

The Hippocratic Oath states in full,

I swear by Apollo the physician and Aesculapius and health and all heal, (that is by Hygieia and Panacea) and all the Gods and Goddesses, that according to my ability and judgement I will keep this oath and this stipulation to reckon him who taught me this Art equally dear to me as my Parents, to share my substance with him and relieve his necessities if required, to look upon his offspring in the same footing as my own brothers, and to teach them this Art if they shall wish to learn it, without fee or stipulation. And that by precept, lecture and every other mode of Instruction, I will impart a knowledge of the Art to my own Sons, and those of my Teachers, and to Disciples bound by a stipulation and Oath according to the Law of Medicine. But to none others. I will follow that system of regimen, which according to my Ability and Judgement, I consider for the benefit of my patients, and abstain from whatever is deleterious and mischievous. I will give no deadly Medicine to anyone if asked, nor suggest any such Counsel. And in like manner I will not give to a Woman a Pessary to procure Abortion. With Purity and with Holiness I will pass my life and practise my Art. I will not cut persons labouring under the stone but will leave this to be done by Men who are Practitioners of this work. Into whatever houses I enter I will go into them for the benefit of the sick, and will abstain from every voluntary act of mischief and corruption, and further from the Seduction of Females or Males of Freemen and Slaves. Whatever, in connection with my professional practice or not in connection with it, I see or hear in the life of men which ought not to be spoken of abroad, I will not divulge, as reckoning that all such should be kept secret. While I continue to keep this Oath unviolated, may it be granted to me to enjoy life and the practice of the Art, respected by all men in all times. But should I trespass and violate this Oath, may the reverse be my lot.

The oath begins "I swear by Apollo." Apollo was god of the sun and god of the intellect and is associated with two basic Greek precepts which every migraine sufferer would do well to reflect upon. These are "Know thyself" and "Nothing in excess." Greek culture respected the value of the individual in society and it is this basic understanding of human nature that makes so many of the writings of the philosophers of ancient Greece as applicable now as they were in their own day.

We often have people complaining that things are not what they were. Naturally enough it is usually members of the older generation who look back wistfully into the past. An obvious target of criticism is the young. Needless to say the young are seldom such splendid products as their critics recall themselves to have been in their own youth. Would it surprise you if one of your friends commented:

> Our youth loves luxury, has bad manners, disregards authority and has no respect whatever for age; today's children are tyrants, they do not get up when an elderly man enters the room, they talk back to their parents.

You are unlikely to be astonished. Probably the friends of Socrates were not surprised either when he aired these views four hundred years before the birth of Christ.

Like youth at the time of Socrates the medical profession of today has not escaped the criticism that things are not what they were. This comment merits some thought in order to discover what relevance, if any, it might have to the treatment of migraine. If a patient calls his doctor because he has a stabbing pain in his chest when he breathes, and is coughing up bloodstained phlegm, the doctor has little difficulty in diagnosing pneumonia with pleurisy. Only thirty years ago pneumonia was an illness in which devoted nursing played a major role in assisting recovery. Today,

129

the physician is armed with a powerful range of antibiotics with which to tackle the problem.

Inevitably, and somewhat regrettably, the relationship between patient and doctor has changed correspondingly. Gone are the days when the doctor called three times a day to see whether little Jimmie was pulling through the complications of measles. Now the doctor prescribes a course of tablets in the sure knowledge that all is likely to be well. Of course one would not want to turn the clock back but one may feel saddened that the improved practice of medical treatment has resulted in a loss of the close familiarity which used to exist between the doctor and his patients. We should not, however, make unfair generalizations as the matter of personal relationships must always remain one for the individuals concerned.

Migraine is a disorder in which this personal contact between doctor and patient is of prime importance. It may not be essential for the surgeon to understand the mode of life of the patient whose appendix he is removing but in treating a patient with a condition like migraine, where the causes are so various, a depth of insight into the physical and mental well-being of the sufferer is vital.

But before we consider the treatment of migraine today let us take one more glance into the past. The first complete and illustrated book on Surgery and Instruments was written by Albucasis, an Arabian Surgeon, who died in A.D. 1013. A beautifully produced definitive edition of the Arabic text with an English translation by Dr. M. S. Spink and Dr. G. L. Lewis has recently been published by the Wellcome Institute of the History of Medicine. The method described by Albucasis for the relief of migraine evoke thoughts of torture rather than treatment. But let me quote from this monumental translation of Albucasis and you can judge for yourselves.

> When there occurs pain with headache in one side of the head and the pain extends to the eye; and the patient has cleared his head with purging drugs and there has been applied the other treatment that I have mentioned in the sections on diseases, but to no avail; in this disorder cauterization is of two sorts, either with caustic or with the actual cautery. This is the manner of cauterization with caustic : take one clove of garlic; peel it and cut both ends off; then cut open the site of the pain in the temple with a broad scalpel till there is room to contain the clove

under the skin; then introduce it under the skin till it lies completely hidden. Then bind up the wound tightly over it with pads and leave for fifteen hours; then unbind it, remove the garlic, and leave the wound open for two or three days; then apply cotton wool soaked in butter till it suppurates. Then dress with ointment till it heals. . . .

The actual cauterization with iron should be done in this way : heat a cautery of this shape. It is called the claviform; the head is nail-shaped in that there is a slight curvature with a small protuberance in the middle. Apply it then to the site of the pain, hold your hand steady and revolve it little by little. Let the thickness of skin burnt be about half; then remove your hand so as not to burn a subjacent artery, for thus a haemorrhage arises. Then soak some cotton wool in saline, apply to the place, and leave three days; then apply cotton wool with butter; then treat with ointment till it heals. Or if you prefer you can cauterize this migraine with the knife-edge that juts out from the cautery, but be careful not to cut an artery, specially in this kind of migraine that is non-chronic.

When you have treated a migraine in the way we have described and with what we have mentioned in the sections on diseases, and the treatment is ineffective, and you perceive that the malady is such that the cauterization we have mentioned before does not suffice for it, either with caustic or with the actual artery, you should heat an edged cautery to white heat after you have marked the place with a line half a finger's breadth long or thereabouts; and impress your hand once and maintain the pressure till you cut down upon the artery and reach the bone. You must be careful of the mandibular joint which moves in chewing, that you do not cut the muscle or tendon that moves it, causing spasm. Have the utmost care of haemorrhage from the artery you have cut, for the occurrence of that is dangerous, specially with one who does not know what to do, having no experience or practice; it is better to refrain from operating. We shall later on mention a treatment for accidental haemorrhage of the artery, in due detail, in its proper place in this book. But if you see that this cautery is not enough for this disorder and you see that the patient is of bodily fitness for it, cauterize him in the middle of the head as we have described, and treat the wound till healed.

The author mentions that Hippocrates advocated bleeding for chronic headache and that Celsus who gave us the classic description of inflammation also described cauterization of the temporal veins.

When the measures already described by Albucasis failed

extraction of the temporal arteries was recommended. This was undertaken as follows:

> The manner of extraction is for the patient to shave the temporal hair; then you press upon the artery appearing on the temple; for it will be manifest to you by its pulsation, and is rarely invisible save in a few people or on account of severe cold. But if it is not plain to you then let the patient bind his neck with the end of his garment; then do you rub the place with a piece of cloth or foment with hot water, till the artery is obvious to you; then take a scalpel shaped thus then with it gently scrape away the skin till you come to the artery, then stick a hook in it and draw it upward till you extract it from the skin and free it all round from the membranes that are beneath it. But if the artery be thin, twist it with the tip of the hook and cut out enough of it for the two ends to be well separated from one another and contract so that no haemorrhage occurs; for if it is not divided and cut it will not let blood flow at all. Then let blood, from six to three ounces.

Bleeding from veins was also undertaken and provides us with our last graphic description taken from the translation of Albucasis.

> Venesection of the two veins behind the ears. Bleeding from both of these will give relief in cases of chronic catarrh, migraine and chronic foul pustules, and scabs of the head. The method of venesecting these two is as I shall now describe: the patient's head should be shaved and the hinder part, in the region of the two veins, should be strongly chafed with a rough cloth; then the patient should bind his neck with his turban until the two veins are visible; their position is behind the ears in the two flattened places of the head; feel for them with your fingers and when you feel their pulsation beneath your finger then mark the place with ink. Then take a knife scalpel, known as a lancet, and insert it beneath the vessel into the skin until the scalpel reaches the bone; then lifting with your hand both vessel and skin make an incision dividing both skin and vein; the length of the incision should be about two fingers side by side; then draw off the quantity of blood you wish. Then bind them up with dressings and leave it until healed.

The fact that patients were prepared to undergo such drastic treatment is some indication of the suffering from which they were seeking relief. Fortunately the passing of a thousand years has provided us with less violent remedies.

If we think about the chief causes of migraine we can list them as follows:

Stress
Hormonal factors
Hunger producing a low blood sugar
Dietary factors

These are discussed individually in various sections of this book. In this particular section we are dealing solely with aspects of drug therapy in migraine. As the exact cause of migraine remains unknown no treatment can be considered curative but we can divide the treatments in current use into those that are aimed at the prophylaxis or prevention of migraine and those that attempt to relieve the symptoms of an attack.

PROPHYLACTIC THERAPY

Sedatives

Probably the most commonly cited precipitant of migraine attacks is stress.

It is not always possible to avoid occasions which cause stress and for this reason the use of a mild sedative is occasionally helpful to the migraine sufferer. If you know that you are going to get very anxious about an interview, or that you will find a particular journey worrying it will probably make all the difference if you take the edge off it with the help of a tablet from your doctor. Of course it would be quite wrong to rely on sedatives as a routine aid to daily living but to illustrate the point, the old proverb of a stitch in time saves nine, might well be translated into a medical context. Some of the drugs used specifically for the prophylaxis of migraine contain a mild sedative for this reason.

Hormone Therapy

Migraine reaches its peak incidence of over ten per cent in the female population between the ages of twenty and forty-five years. This is undoubtedly related to the increased frequency of migraine at certain stages in the menstrual cycle. A chart recording the dates on which headaches occur and the times of menstruation over a length of time covering three months or more may prove very helpful. The normal menstrual cycle lasts twenty-eight days and where attacks occur most often in the middle of this cycle, or during or immediately after a menstrual period it is probable that the symptoms are related to changes in the oestrogen level in the blood. These are times when the oestrogen levels are relatively high.

Occasionally patients are given treatment with oestrogens for such conditions as hot flushes. These patients sometimes report an increase in the severity of their headaches. Migrainous headaches occurring for the first time have also been reported in patients on oestrogen therapy.

A number of women notice that they seem to store water in their bodies before they develop an attack of migraine. The rings on their fingers, the waistbands of their skirts and their shoes may all feel tighter than usual. Oestrogen therapy sometimes produces water retention and the water retention which occurs naturally during certain phases of the menstrual cycle may reflect a rise in oestrogen levels in the body. This water retention is often noticed in the middle of the menstrual cycle or just before the onset of a menstrual period.

During the second half of the hormonal cycle when the incidence of headaches is less frequent, the hormone progesterone is being secreted. This has led to the use of progesterone as a treatment for women who suffer from migraine headaches bearing a clear relation to the menstrual cycle. The response to progesterone appears to be particularly good in those patients whose attacks occur just before or during menstruation.

Progesterone can be given either by intramuscular injection or in suppository form. When prescribed by injection the dose is twenty-five to fifty milligrams on alternate days during the second half of the menstrual cycle. Alternatively progesterone suppositories can be given in doses varying from fifty to four hundred milligrams a day.

Progesterone therapy is worth trying in patients with menopausal migraine and in any patient in whom hormonal factors might play a role.

Methysergide Therapy

Normal blood contains a substance called 5-hydroxytryptamine (serotonin). At the onset of a migraine attack the level of this substance falls to about forty per cent of its usual level. The role of serotonin in migraine has been extensively investigated and about eighty per cent of migraine sufferers investigated have shown this drop in serotonin levels at the onset of an attack. It seems reasonable, therefore, to assume that a change in serotonin levels is a feature of migraine attacks.

About ten years ago, soon after it was established that the levels of serotonin in the blood played a role in the migraine attack, the drug methysergide was introduced into migraine therapy. Methysergide acts as a powerful antagonist of serotonin and has proved to be an effective preventive treatment in migraine. It lessens the frequency and the severity of attacks in well over half the sufferers in whom it has been used.

Unfortunately, however, there are snags. Methysergide is not without possible harmful effects. These usually begin to occur after treatment with the drug has been given for several weeks and the incidence is thought to be about forty per cent. All drugs have certain toxic effects in common and these, as one might expect, are nausea, vomiting and diarrhoea. Skin rashes are also a common toxic effect of most drugs. These relatively mild toxic side effects may be accompanied by nervousness and insomnia in patients on methysergide treatment. The mild mental effects produced occasionally may have some bearing on the fact that methysergide is chemically related to the psychotropic drug LSD. About fifteen per cent of the patients on methysergide therapy have to discontinue treatment with the drug because of these side effects.

Methysergide, however, can produce another very much rarer but much more serious side effect. This is a thickening of the tissues in the back of the abdominal wall. This can involve veins in the area and also put pressure on the ureters which are the narrow tubes which carry urine from the kidneys to the bladder. The condition is a low grade inflammation and is termed "retroperitoneal fibrosis." The patient who develops this complication may complain of a low backache. Swelling of one leg may be an early sign resulting from pressure from the thickened tissues on the veins carrying blood from the legs. In other patients a slight rise in temperature may occur and a diminished output in the daily amount of urine may be noticed.

Migraine

As the toxic effects of methysergide do not usually occur until the drug has been used for several weeks, methysergide therapy is usually prescribed on an intermittent basis. If any side effects show themselves the drug is stopped immediately and any damage done is usually reversible. When a patient has been treated with the drug for a period of six months then therapy is interrupted for a period of at least six weeks.

Methysergide is made up in tablets containing two milligrams of the drug. The highest daily dose which can be taken is four tablets but fewer are advisable if satisfactory results can be obtained with less than a total of eight milligrams daily.

During an attack of migraine the branches of the external carotid artery become enlarged and distended. Work on methysergide has shown that it causes a very marked decrease in the blood flow of the external carotid artery circulation. Possibly methysergide is such an effective prophylactic therapy for migraine because it prevents the vascular dilation which is associated with the onset of pain in migraine.

Dixarit Therapy

This is a relatively new drug which was introduced into the treatment of migraine in 1969. Its major advantage is that it has no known harmful effects. In considering the use of any treatment with drugs one has to weigh the possible harmful effects of the drug against the benefits that one hopes will arise from it. When there is any doubt about it, it is best not to use the drug. One would not, for example, consider using methysergide for a patient with migraine unless the attacks were frequent and severe. Dixarit, like methysergide, is used as a preventive treatment. It appears to benefit about sixty to seventy per cent of patients. Although they may still suffer from headaches, these headaches become less frequent and less severe, and more amenable to analgesic therapy if they occur. The drug appears to be particularly helpful to patients who associate some of their attacks with the eating of certain foods such as chocolate, cheese, alcohol and citrus fruits. Some of these foods contain amines like tyramine and beta-phenylethylamine which have an effect on blood vessels and provoke a headache in a proportion of migraine sufferers. About one in three migraine subjects respond to dietary factors in this way. Dixarit acts by reducing the sensitivity or reactivity of blood vessels to any sort of stimuli and this is the basis on which it was introduced to migraine therapy.

It is of interest that Dixarit has also been found useful in treating the hot flushes that occasionally prove an embarrassment to women during the menopause. This is hardly surprising when one considers that flushing is due to an overactivity of blood vessels.

Dixarit tablets contain twenty-five micrograms of clonidine hydrochloride. It has been found that clonidine in doses of one to two micrograms per kilogram of body weight decreases the response of peripheral blood vessels to any stimuli. This means that the blood vessels so treated do not dilate or constrict as much as normal. Dixarit tablets are bright blue. A starting dose is one tablet twice a day but the dosage can be gradually increased up to about six, or even in some patients to eight a day. The tablets should be spread as evenly as possible throughout the waking hours of the day. Larger doses than eight a day could have an effect in lowering the blood pressure. Considerably larger doses of clonidine hydrochloride are contained in the drug Catapres, which is used in the treatment of high blood pressure.

The length of time for which a patient should stay on Dixarit treatment varies. Sometimes the dose has to be stepped up gradually until an effective level of anything up to eight tablets a day is reached. The maximum benefit from Dixarit is not always obtained before treatment has continued for up to three months and in doubtful cases it is well worthwhile continuing therapy for at least this length of time. Improvement is often dramatic and when it has been maintained for a few months it is worth tapering off Dixarit therapy gradually to see whether the improvement continues without the drug. Treatment can always be restarted again if needed.

Dixarit is the only specific therapy for migraine which is not derived from the alkaloids of ergot. Patients taking Dixarit do not suffer from the side effects which make ergot a drug to be used with great caution.

Some patients on Dixarit complain of drowsiness. When this is severe it is worth trying the effect of two Dixarit tablets only at night. Dryness of the mouth occasionally occurs but usually passes off after a few weeks. Dizziness, nausea and restlessness at night have also been reported. Skin rashes are a common manifestation of treatment with most drugs if toxic symptoms arise.

The only patients in whom Dixarit should not be used are those who have a history of depressive illness. Occasionally Dixarit makes these symptoms worse. Depression in a migraine patient is difficult to judge. Anyone who suffered from constant, recurring thumping headaches might well get depressed. In such patients the relief which might accompany Dixarit therapy could well alter the sufferer's mental state.

The tragic thalidomide disaster has increased our awareness of the possible harmful effects of drugs on the unborn child. Extensive testing of pregnant animals has not shown Dixarit to have any harmful effects on the developing foetus. It is probably best, however, to avoid Dixarit during the first three months of pregnancy as this is the time when the developing foetus is most susceptible to harmful influences. In fact, all but absolutely essential therapy would best be avoided at this time.

Migraine not uncommonly occurs in patients with a slightly raised blood pressure. These patients usually benefit from larger doses of the drug. Dixarit should not be used in migraine sufferers who are already receiving other treatment for a high blood pressure.

Anticonvulsant Drugs

These drugs are usually prescribed for the treatment of epilepsy. They are sometimes of help to migraine sufferers especially in those in whom an electroencephalogram reveals unusual activity at the surface of the brain. It is this group of migraine patients who probably benefit most from anticonvulsant drugs such as phenytoin. They have been found of particular help in younger migraine patients and are usually used in small doses over a long period of time.

Needless to say, time is not the major factor in prophylactic treatment and most of the drugs used for the prevention of migraine attacks can be given by mouth. One exception is hormone therapy with progesterone which must be given either by intramuscular injection or in suppository form.

Before we pass on to the treatment of the acute attack of migraine we can make a pause and consider how migraine used to be treated one hundred years ago.

In 1870, a physician, J. Waring Curran, wrote :

> In most of these cases considered hemicrania treated by myself, I have exhausted the Pharmacopoeia. Some patients had large quantities of quinine, others liquor arsenicalis without much benefit or marked effect. My great objection to the two sheet anchors, quinine and arsenic are that in most of the cases, after a few days we have derangement of stomach, so that both remedies mentioned are objectionable, accordingly I have given salicin with more satisfaction than any other remedy.

Salicin is a substance which is in the same group of substances as aspirin. It is less efficient than aspirin and often produces skin rashes. It is now no longer used.

Another remedy which was strongly advocated about one hundred years ago is described in the words of an article in the Boston Medical and Surgical Journal in 1879 written by Dr. S. Weir Mitchell. The patient is a lady who is recommended to take the following measures :

> When the attack comes on she is to lie down in a darkened and quiet room. Cold applications to the head and a mustard foot bath might be useful adjuncts to the treatment.
> I may add that the use of the old domestic remedy, a tight bandage during the attack is useful. I make use of a rubber bandage, applied thoroughly from the eyes up with a thin pad over each temporal artery, if the temporal ridge be sharp enough to keep the bandage from squeezing the arteries, and over the two occipital vessels. Instead of a caoutchouc, a well applied muslin bandage may be put on and then wetted, using compresses over the temporal arteries. The comfort thus given is sometimes surprising. I need not say that migraine in some of its forms becomes at times, and in women especially, a most disabling malady, and may recur daily until life is a burden impatiently borne. These are usually cases of thin blooded and thin people, whose sufferings are brought back by the attempt to take exercise, without an abundance of which a return to health is out of the question. I have seen some such cases in which a cure little less than marvellous has been made by the use of absolute rest, overfeeding and massage. There is, of course, much more to be said on the therapeutics of megrims, but no one drug is its master. The hint as to thorough bandaging is worth remembering and especially at the close of a headache.

The use of tight bandages is no longer advocated as a treatment today, but it is a well-known fact to many migraine sufferers

Migraine

in the throes of an acute attack that pressing the affected side of
the head into a pillow produces some relief.

TREATMENT OF AN ATTACK

Time is a factor of major importance when the symptoms of
migraine begin to make themselves felt. Once the headache has
really developed there is little the sufferer can do to ease it to
any great degree. There are four main ways in which drugs can
be given for migraine.

By mouth
By inhalation
In suppository form
By intramuscular injection.

A tablet taken by mouth can either be swallowed immediately
or kept under the tongue while it dissolves. Everyone is aware of
the way in which people who get angina when they exert themselves put a nitroglycerine tablet under their tongues and rest
while it slowly dissolves with relief of the pain. A new ergot compound which can be taken in this way for migraine has recently
become available.

The classical remedy for migraine is rest in a darkened room
with or without a pot of strong black coffee at the bedside. How
delightful, if anything can appear delightful at that stage, the
prospect of rest in a darkened room appears to the migraine
sufferer in the throes of an acute attack. Usually the unfortunate
victim has just to struggle home from work or is unable to get
to bed because the needs of small children cannot be ignored.
Every migraine sufferer knows the bliss of finally burying that
pounding head in a pillow. No, rest in a darkened room may be
the ideal solution, but circumstances are seldom ideal. So what
does one do?

Analgesics

Aspirin remains the most commonly and effectively used
therapy for a migraine attack. There are many analgesic tablets
on the market containing such substances as aspirin, codeine,
paracetamol and phenacetin. Thousand of tons of these analgesic
tablets are consumed every year despite the fact that they are

not without their harmful side effects. Aspirin in large doses can cause nausea, vomiting, diarrhoea, skin rashes, buzzing in the ears and giddiness. Aspirin also irritates the lining of the stomach and can occasionally produce ulceration and bleeding from the stomach. Phenacetin used to be a common ingredient in headache relieving powders and tablets. It is still found in some compounds, but should be avoided, as prolonged or excessive use can result in long lasting ill effects particularly on the kidneys. Codeine is also contained in a number of compounds. It tends to have a constipating effect. Paracetamol is commonly used and as it does not cause gastric irritation it is an analgesic that is often preferred to aspirin. All analgesic tablets should be taken with fluid in order to minimize their effect on the lining of the stomach. If you want to see what happens in your stomach when you take an aspirin tablet you can try keeping one between your gum and your cheek while it dissolves. A raw inflamed area is likely to result. So even household remedies like aspirin should not be taken without due care. Furthermore prolonged and excessive use of analgesics can result in an almost continuous headache. Obviously if you feel a headache coming on you have got to take something to try and prevent it developing or to reduce its severity. The warning about analgesics is not intended to deter headache sufferers from taking them *in moderation* when absolutely necessary, but to draw attention to the fact that they can have harmful effects and should not be taken routinely like food.

Aspirin and other commonly used analgesics such as paracetamol and codeine are the treatment of choice in people who suffer from common migraine. Phenacetin is best avoided in view of the kidney damage it is thought capable of causing.

Classical migraine is differentiated from common migraine by the fact that the attack is heralded by an aura or warning signs. These signs are usually visual. The most effective drug therapy for classical migraine is ergot. Many peole with common migraine also use drugs containing ergot and find them beneficial.

Ergot

Ergot is obtained from the fungus *Claviceps purpurea*. This fungus is a parasite which grows on a number of grasses. Ergot, however, is usually obtained from rye. Ergot contains a number of alkaloids of which the most important are ergonovine, ergo-toscine and ergotamine.

In the past chronic poisoning with ergot occurred frequently in people fed on rye that was infected with the fungus. A village baker could be responsible for poisoning a whole community and the suffering must have been severe. Ergot poisoning was probably the cause of the great plague of Athens in the fifth century before Christ. The symptoms of ergot poisoning include burning and tingling in the hands and feet. For this reason it used to be called St. Anthony's fire. The name derived from the Saint to whom supplications for relief were made. Ergot poisoning could result in peripheral gangrene with resultant gross deformity and loss of the extremities. The last known epidemic of ergotism was in 1816 but sporadic cases are still reported from time to time and can result from therapy with ergot compounds.

Ergot has no effect whatever when it is applied externally to the body. When it is given internally it has a powerful effect on the muscle of the pregnant womb. For this reason it used to be a common ingredient of substances employed to procure abortions. For this reason also ergot should never be prescribed for migraine during pregnancy.

It is nevertheless this action of ergot on the uterus which has provided its chief benefit to mankind in general and women in particular. An injection of an ergot compound is standard practice during the third stage of childbirth. During the first stage the womb prepares to expel the child and the cervical canal through which the baby has to pass gradually dilates. At the end of the second stage the baby is born. It is attached to the mother by the umbilical cord which connects the baby to the placenta. This is a fleshy pad through which the developing embryo derives all its food and nourishment. The placenta is expelled during the third stage of labour leaving behind it a raw surface. The muscle of the womb contracts to stop this raw area from bleeding excessively and this contraction is assisted very greatly by an injection of ergometrine maleate which is given intra-muscularly during the third stage of labour.

Ergot also has a direct action on blood vessels and causes them to constrict. It is this constricting action of ergot which sometimes results in peripheral gangrene in the limbs.

The ergot compound which is used most commonly in migraine

is ergotamine. This was isolated from ergot in 1918. The blood
vessels in the painful area of the head during a migraine attack
are enlarged and painful and it is the constricting action of ergot
which reduces the size of these vessels and relieves the pain.

Ergot can be given in four different ways, by mouth, by inhalation, by injection and in suppository form. If ergot is to be helpful it should be taken as soon as the patient feels that an attack
is inevitable. If a patient is feeling sick and vomiting it is obviously useless taking ergotamine tablets by mouth. Some people
cannot bear the thought of sticking a needle into themselves and
they would obviously avoid ergot by injection. Suppositories
provide the answer for a large number of sufferers but the route
of administration chosen by an individual obviously depends on
various factors.

Ergotamine abuse is very common. Some migraine sufferers
make an almost daily habit of using it. Despite warnings about
the dangers of excessive ergot administration, these sufferers consider that they cannot do without it. They try to justify this by
complaining that their headaches keep recurring without realizing that the reason why they keep recurring is their constant use
of ergotamine. Ergot abuse results in a vicious cycle of headaches.
Prolonged ergot therapy can produce a paralysis of the nerves
which supply the blood vessels and the latter stages in a migraine
sufferer may be worse than the first. The headache becomes
continuous.

Ergot can also produce other unwelcome side effects. The first
symptoms of poisoning usually occur in the circulatory system.
The sufferer may notice that he is always feeling chilly and
cramps may cause trouble in the legs. A feeling of nausea may
become marked and occasionally vomiting and diarrhoea, which
are common side effects of a large number of drugs, occur.
Patients taking too much ergot sometimes notice tingling in their
hands and feet. All these side effects provide a warning that
should not be ignored and ergot therapy should be stopped at
once if they occur.

Small doses of ergotamine are more effective in producing
headache relief than large doses. The drug should be taken as
early as possible in an attack.

Ergotamine tartrate is prepared in the following forms for the
treatment of migraine.

Tablets. These are taken by mouth. A new tablet is available which does not have to be swallowed but can be held under the tongue until it dissolves. The dose of ergotamine tartrate contained in each tablet is one milligram. One tablet should be taken at the onset of the attack and this can be repeated in an hour if necessary. Not more than four tablets should be taken in twenty-four hours and not more than eight tablets in a week.

Suppositories. Ergotamine suppositories contain two milligrams of ergotamine tartrate each. They often contain caffeine in addition as this is thought to enhance the effect of ergotamine. This is a particularly successful method of treating attacks in which the patient feels sick and is vomiting. One suppository should be used at the beginning of an attack and a further suppository can be used after about an hour if needed. No more than three suppositories should be used in a day or five in a week. If a whole suppository is effective it is worth seeing whether a half will be effective in view of the benefits of decreasing the amount of ergot taken.

By Inhalation. Ergotamine can also be taken by inhalation. The Medihaler ergotamine contains 0.36 milligrams of ergotamine per puff or per inhalation. Migraine sufferers are advised to take one inhalation as soon as possible after the onset of an attack and to repeat this, if needed, at intervals of ten minutes for a maximum of five inhalations or puffs.

By Injection. Ergotamine tartrate injections contain 0.25 milligrams of ergotamine tartrate. They are given subcutaneously or intramuscularly. They can be repeated once only during an attack if necessary. No more than a maximum of four injections should be given during any one week.

There are a number of migraine sufferers who exceed the advisable limits of therapy with ergot. Very often these are the patients who have developed a cycle of incessant headaches as a result of ergot toxicity. These patients should seek the help of their doctors. A short spell in hospital is sometimes helpful to these sufferers while they are weaned on to less harmful treatment.

Treatment with ergot has been discussed at length. The reasons for this are obvious as it is a drug to which many migraine sufferers readily resort without always realizing fully its potential for harm.

It was emphasized previously that the most commonly used therapy for an acute attack of migraine is aspirin and other ordinary analgesics. This section would not be complete, however, without at least a brief mention of one or two other methods by which an acute attack has been tackled.

Indomethacin Therapy

Indomethacin is an analgesic, anti-inflammatory and anti-pyretic drug which is usually used for the treatment of arthritic conditions and gout. Despite the fact that one of its side effects may be headache, it has been tried in the treatment of an acute attack of migraine and has apparently been helpful to some patients. The dose is in suppository form: 100 milligrams at the onset of an attack then 25 milligrams capsules by mouth every four hours up to a total dose of four tablets. Indomethacin should not be tried in any patient suffering from a peptic ulcer.

Dixarit Therapy

This is being tried in the treatment of an acute attack of migraine. Where a warning of an impending attack occurs in patients who are taking Dixarit as a prophylactic therapy it is often helpful to take one or two extra tablets at once. Patients not on Dixarit therapy who feel that an attack is coming on should try to see whether or not the taking of one or two Dixarit tablets either averts the attack or reduces its usual severity. Dixarit appears to be a help to a number of migraine sufferers when it is taken in this way. In any case it is well worth giving it a trial in view of the lack of toxic effects.

Patients who are on prophylactic therapy with Dixarit often find that simple measures like aspirin are more effective than they used to be in alleviating their headaches when they occur.

TREATMENT IN CHILDREN

Migraine in very young children is so rare as to be relatively unknown. By the age of five the incidence of migraine is one per cent. By the age of eleven it has risen to five per cent.

The most important thing to do in children with headaches

Migraine

is to make sure that the diagnosis is correct. If a mother suffers from migraine herself and her child starts having headaches she should let a doctor see the child and decide upon the treatment. It would be quite wrong if the parents assumed the child had migraine, like its mother, and failed to get treatment for some other cause of the pain, such as ear or tooth trouble, which was then neglected. So the first essential in treating a child with migraine is to ensure that a correct diagnosis is made. Powerful drugs like ergot should not be used in children.

Very often a mild sedative such as phenobarbitone for a few weeks is all that is needed to reduce the frequency and severity of the headaches. Where further treatment is necessary ordinary analgesics such as soluble aspirin are the best way to tackle the problem when a headache begins. It is vital to give the analgesic as soon as possible. Trouble sometimes arises with children at school who develop a headache during school hours. They may be too shy to explain to the teacher that they are getting a headache and several hours can pass before they get home. By then it is too late for any tablets to be effective. For this reason it is a good idea for the mother of a child with migraine to speak to the teacher and explain the position. The child can then take a suitable tablet to school and be encouraged to take it as soon as a headache begins.

OTHER FORMS OF TREATMENT

Anti-emetics

Nausea and vomiting and the dizziness which often accompanies these symptoms are common features of an attack of migraine. For this reason anti-emetic drugs are often included in the proprietary preparations specifically prepared for the migraine sufferer.

Some migraine patients suffer from severe dizziness during an attack. This dizziness may in fact be the major symptom in a small proportion of patients. It can be treated with drugs used specifically for vertigo or dizziness.

Prostaglandins and Migraine

Relatively recently a new group of substances called prostaglandins have appeared on the medical scene. It seems to be highly likely that these prostaglandins are concerned in the production of inflammation and of pain. It is therefore of interest when we think about methods of relieving pain in migraine that aspirin and indomethacin are known to inhibit the production of prostaglandins.

Migraine and Acupuncture

The subject of acupuncture has aroused increasing interest in Britain. Devised by the Chinese as a method of treatment many centuries before the birth of Christ it has stood the test of centuries of time. We do not understand how it works in the relief of pain and it puzzles and fascinates us as a method that is foreign to our way of thinking. Chinese medicine differs from our own because it is founded on ancient philosophical concepts. This is far removed from the mathematical logic and experimental observation on which our modern scientific medicine is based.

In the last twenty-five years the practise of acupuncture has increased in the Western world. It is used particularly in France and Germany. An International Institute of Acupuncture has been formed and there is also a French Institute of Acupuncture. The subject of Acupuncture is recognized by the Faculty of Medicine in Paris.

Another term for acupuncture is needling, which tells us in one word what it is about. Acupuncture is performed by the use of needles. Traditionally these needles were of nine kinds, arrow headed, blunt, puncturing, spearpointed, ensiform, round, capillary, long and great. They were made of steel, copper or silver with brass wire handles. The needles were inserted into the flesh at depths and sites varying with the condition to be treated. Sometimes a light blow from a mallet was necessary in order to insert the needle. The needles were used either hot or cold. If heating was required then herbs were placed around the brass wire at the end of the needle and ignited. The needles were left in position for varying lengths of time. They might be left for a few minutes or for much longer periods, even up to days on end.

The technique of acupuncture was derived from the ancient Chinese philosophical concept of opposing forces in nature. Everything was related to the elements, the planets, the seasons and the time of day. Everything possessed the qualities of Yang and Yin in varying proportions. The idea of Yang was associated with light, the sun, the south and with maleness. The idea of Yin was associated with darkness, the moon, the north and femaleness. In order to lead a good life and to maintain health a perfect balance between Yang and Yin was necessary. If this

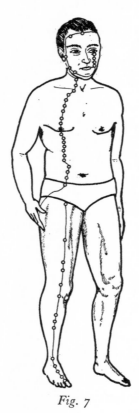

Fig. 7

balance was disturbed in a human being disease resulted and the method of acupuncture was devised as a means of restoring harmony between the opposing forces of Yin and Yang.

According to Chinese tradition the contrasting components Yin and Yang are carried in a series of separate channels in the human body. These channels are called meridians. Models of the human body showing these meridians and acupuncture points are made and date from ancient times (see Figure 7). The acupuncture points lie either on the meridians or at their intersections. Traditionally there are 365 acupuncture points along twelve meridians. The site chosen for acupuncture is related only in an empirical way to the area in which pain is to be relieved. The time at which acupuncture may be performed in Chinese medicine is closely related to the seasons and time of the month. For example, on the third day of the month acupuncture of the thigh was forbidden. On the sixteenth day acupuncture of the chest was forbidden.

This approach to therapy may seem strange to our Western minds but there is no doubt that acupuncture can be a successful method of relieving pain. The fact that we do not understand why or how this takes place does not alter the fact that it can be a highly successful therapy.

During the process of acupuncture, while the needles are in position, a constant stimulation of the tissues is undertaken. Either the needles are constantly twirled around by hand, or they are heated by the burning of herbs. Nowadays an electric current may be passed between two needles. The relief of pain or production of anaesthesia may develop very slowly. Anaesthesia sometimes lasts for several hours after the needles are withdrawn. The use of acupuncture as a means of inducing anaesthesia in surgery is of particular interest. The needles may be inserted at some distance from the site of operation. For example the removal of a stomach may be undertaken under anaesthesia produced by the insertion of four acupuncture needles in the lobes of the ear.

Acupuncture was one of the chief methods available to a Chinese physician. Confucius (551–479 B.C.) objected strongly to the dissection of the human body after death or any cutting of the body in life. Surgery, therefore, could not develop under the Chinese system.

Some sceptics dismiss acupuncture as a form of hypnosis or autosuggestion. Doubtless faith on the part of the patient plays an integral part in the success of the method and the Chinese belief in acupuncture is based on the tradition of many centuries. Only about one in five people respond to hypnotism and the success rate with acupuncture is considerably higher than this which leaves one wondering by what other means the technique of acupuncture produces its effects.

Acupuncture has been used chiefly in the treatment of such conditions as headache, convulsions and arthritis. In the section of this book on the causes of migraine attention was focused on the role of the autonomic nervous system in the control of blood vessels. When the two parts of the autonomic nervous system, the sympathetic and parasympathetic systems were first described they were likened to the opposing forces of Yang and Yin. If we extend this parallel further it might lead us to suggest that conditions such as migraine are precisely those which might benefit most from acupuncture therapy.

It is a fact that one in four migraine sufferers is likely to benefit from almost any new therapy, at least for a while. One would therefore anticipate that if all migraine sufferers were given treatment by acupuncture about one quarter of them would report an improvement in their symptoms. It is difficult to see how one could ever undertake a controlled investigation into the efficacy of acupuncture in migraine and the facts will gradually have to speak for themselves. This will take time; if enough migraine sufferers decide to try acupuncture we shall slowly be able to collect our evidence. In the meantime, or rather at the same time, further investigations and new theories of pain may eventually explain why the method is so often successful.

We accept that any measure which is of psychological benefit and relieves stress is likely to help a proportion of migraine sufferers. This is probably why hypnosis sometimes proves to be so effective. Other factors may also contribute to the success of acupuncture but time alone will tell us what they are.

18

Attending a Migraine Clinic

MANY sufferers from migraine are unaware that special clinics exist up and down the country for the treatment of this disorder. Others know about these clinics but hesitate to attend them. They may have put up with their headaches for many years and do not feel like making what they consider might be a fuss about them now. Others are worried about what might happen to them if they do go to a clinic and protest in advance that they are not having any needles stuck into them or that "they will only experiment on you if you go there." So what would it be like if you decided to attend a clinic?

You would, of course, have to discuss the matter with your own doctor first. The family doctor is really the ideal doctor to treat migraine because he sees the whole of a patient's background and circumstances. But very often he is glad to send a patient to a migraine clinic to obtain a fresh point of view. The doctor at the clinic will certainly be very pleased to see you as he has chosen to work there because of his particular interest in migraine.

First of all you will be asked for a very careful history of your headaches. This account of your life will go back to the earliest days that you can remember in order to ascertain whether or not you used to suffer from such things as travel sickness or eczema. In fact it will go back even further than your life and ask you to recall whether or not your grandparents or parents suffered from headaches. You may feel that you are unlikely to know what your grandparents did or did not suffer from, but in fact it is usually well known to the other members of a family if someone has one of his or her "heads" repeatedly—and if you were in touch with your grandparents at all and never heard about it then the chances are that none of them had migraine. The careful history will include an account of your habits. Do you smoke? Smoking is thought to increase the incidence of migraine attacks and some people actually relate some of their attacks to being in a smoky atmosphere. Do you drink? You hardly need to be told about the frequent association between migraine attacks and the drinking of alcoholic beverages. This does not by any means prevent large numbers of migraine sufferers from drinking them and then being surprised when they suffer from a headache. Do you eat regular meals? The association between missing a meal and developing a headache has been well authenticated. These and many other questions and answers will piece together the pattern of your life in order to help the doctor in the clinic to discover what triggers off your attacks.

This may take more time than you think, as these factors are not always obvious. For example, a man may get a headache once a week because he plays darts with the boys the night before, misses his usual evening meal and eats a cheese sandwich and bar of chocolate instead. Fortified by a few drinks he arrives home later than usual, happy but overtired. When he wakes in the morning with a thumping head he may be unwilling to associate it with the good time he had a few hours before. A busy housewife may get migraine on a certain day every week because her young son has games that afternoon and announces the fact that he has mislaid his football boots a few minutes before the school bus is due to leave. There are some lessons that some of us never learn from experience. A frenzied search ensues during which everyone gets agitated and upset. It reveals them just in time. This is the day on which she rushes through her housework to have lunch with a friend. This means a wild dash for the train. By the time she arrives at the friend's house and has a hasty meal and a chat it is almost time to rush back to be at home again, before the young man returns from school. The whole day, which is meant to be her one pleasurable day out during the week is one big rush. By evening she is exhausted and it is hardly surprising that she wakes with a headache in the early hours of the following morning.

Now let us return from the different ways in which people inflict well-meaning stresses and strains on themselves to the

peace and quiet of our migraine clinic. You may feel quite prepared for a lot of questions and the usual medical examination.
During this the doctor will listen to your heart and lungs and
check your nervous system. He will also look at your eyes with
an instrument called an ophthalmoscope. A light shines through
your pupil and the back of your eye is seen through a magnifying
lens. At the back of the eye is the retina and a white disc shaped
area which is the optic nerve. The back of the eye is the only
part of the body where one can obtain a direct view of a nerve
and all the arteries and veins which run across the retina. This
examination tells the doctor a great deal both about the state of
the optic nerve and the state of the blood vessels.

But you are still anxious and a little worried because you keep
wondering what sort of investigations you will be asked to undergo. Will anyone try to stick any needles into you?

There are, of course, a certain number of routine tests which
are undertaken on the majority of patients who are attending
an outpatient clinic. One of these is a blood test to check whether
or not you are anaemic or suffering from a hidden infection
which might be contributing to your headaches.

An examination of the urine is also a routine for most patients
attending hospital. It can reveal such conditions as possible
diabetes if sugar is detected, or possible kidney trouble if protein
is found. Both of these conditions can influence the course of
migraine. Sometimes a slight rise in blood pressure can increase
the severity of attacks. This can very easily be treated with great
benefit to the sufferer.

The E.S.R. or erythrocyte sedimentation rate is usually done.
The erythrocytes are red blood cells and this test estimates the
rate at which they settle to the bottom of a narrow glass tube.
The rate is increased in some forms of anaemia and in a number
of acute conditions such as rheumatoid arthritis. It is, also,
markedly raised in one particular type of headache, called
temporal arteritis. This occurs most frequently in people between
the ages of fifty and eighty and the pain affects the temporal
arteries which can be felt beating just in front of the ears. A
raised E.S.R. is an indication that some associated condition
should be sought with the diagnosis of headache.

In some clinics X-rays of the chest and skull are also taken
but this is not always done as a matter of course. As about thirty

per cent of migraine patients show changes in an electroencephalogram this is also sometimes done. The examination is completely harmless, painless and inexpensive. Small electrodes are
placed on the skull at various points and the tiny electrical waves
which they pick up from the activity at the surface of the brain
are recorded.

If the doctor suspects that you might benefit from wearing
spectacles or seeing a dentist you will probably be asked whether
you wish to make your own arrangements for this or attend the
appropriate clinic at the hospital. Eye strain and dental trouble
can both be occasional causes of headache.

These are the more usual investigations carried out in a
migraine clinic. There are other tests which can be helpful in
diagnosing a patient whose headaches do not fit into a typical
pattern. Even these tests would not worry you if they were done,
but if you feel at all nervous about anything you must let the
doctor and staff at the clinic know. They are there to help you
and are well aware of the fact that even the toughest men have
been known to turn pale and faint at the sight of a needle!

19

Sleep

THERE is a story of a professor who during his lecture threw a
piece of chalk at a student and said "If I can keep awake during
this, so can you." Not only was he a bore, but he was inaccurate.
We all know the unpleasant sensation of trying desperately to
keep awake during a dull talk. Sleep overcomes us in the absence
of physical or mental stimulation. This is why people choose a
quiet, darkened room when they want to sleep. All living creatures

have regular periods when they rest and become unaware of their surroundings.

We all have our own preferential sleep pattern. Some of us like to rise with the lark. This state of affairs and the noisy activity that so often accompanies it is incomprehensible, not to say irritating, to the owls among us who only become really alert during the evening hours.

Sleep is necessary to us. It is part of the circadian or twenty-four hour rhythm of our bodies. Certain changes occur during sleep. Our kidneys secrete a more concentrated urine and its volume falls. The level of catecholamine excretion falls to its lowest levels during the early hours of each new day. The tone of our blood vessels changes during sleep. You have only to think of the pink, flushed, refreshed appearance of someone who has just woken from slumber.

Knowing that moderation in all things should be the motto of any migraine sufferer none will be surprised to learn that both too little or too much sleep can be causes of migraine. One or two late nights may be enough to precipitate a headache. Similarly the luxury of an extra hour or two in bed in the morning may lead to a throbbing headache on waking. Sometimes one or two extra pillows are helpful in preventing this especially if these are put under the head at the usual time of waking. A light warm shawl around the head can be helpful. After all the rest of the body is kept warm in bed and only the head is exposed. Many people like to sleep with open windows and howling gales are not unknown in bedrooms. Vascular tone changes with temperature and we know that changes in vascular tone are sometimes associated with the onset of headache. Whatever the merits of keeping a cool head in the decisions of life may be, a comfortably warm head is a good insurance as far as migraine is concerned.

20

Time

"But at my back I always hear
Time's winged chariot hurrying near."
ANDREW MARVELL

TIME waits for no man and who would really wish it to stand still? Even the young and happy look forward constantly to the next new exciting event. Although every stage in life presents its own problems we are spurred on by hope and hope always relates to the future.

The passing of time, however, is not without compensations and for the migraine sufferer these include a marked decrease in the incidence and severity of attacks. Blood vessels slowly become less reactive to stimuli and hormonal activity gradually decreases. Amines are released less readily from body stores. Growing older we might expect to grow a little wiser. As time goes by we should learn, metaphorically speaking, to spend less and less of it in getting headaches through knocking our heads against brick walls.

This book began with a comment on the fact that migraine was recognized over three thousand years ago. Should that make us reflect with sorrow that we are still asking the question "What is migraine?" No, we must look into the future. We must look with the eye of faith. Then we shall see eager historians in times to come turning over dusty pages and murmuring "What *was* migraine?"

Glossary of Terms

ALLERGY   An unusual or exaggerated reaction to a substance.

AMMONIA   A compound containing nitrogen and hydrogen. Formula NH_3.

AMINE   A compound formed from ammonia when one or more of the hydrogen atoms is replaced by organic (hydro carbon) radicals.

AMINO ACID   Compounds containing an amino group (NH_2) and a carboxyl group (COOH). They form the chief structure of proteins.

ANALGESIC   A remedy for pain.

ANTIBIOTIC   A substance which acts against bacteria e.g. penicillin.

AUTONOMIC NERVOUS SYSTEM   Consists of the sympathetic and parasympathetic nervous system and controls involuntary functions.

AURA   A sensation that precedes the onset of a paroxysmal attack.

BETA PHENYLETHYLAMINE   A vasoactive amine found in chocolate, cheese, alcoholic drinks.

CAPILLARIES   Minute vessels which connect the smallest branches of arteries and veins.

CATECHOLAMINES   The hormones produced by the suprarenal glands namely adrenaline and noradrenaline.

CENTRAL NERVOUS SYSTEM   The brain and spinal cord controlling mainly voluntary action.

CIRCADIAN RHYTHM   Biological changes with a cycle of about 24 hours related in some degree to the presence or absence of light.

CEREBRAL   Related to the brain. Extracerebral outside the skull. Intracerebral inside the skull.

ELECTROENCEPHALOGRAM (E.E.G.)   Tracing of the electrical activity of the brain.

ENZYMES   Protein substances present in minute amounts in the body which produce changes in other substances without themselves undergoing any change.

FORTIFICATION SPECTRA   Bizarre lines and shapes seen by some migraine sufferers about 15 minutes before an attack.

GLYCOGEN   The form in which glucose is stored in the liver and in muscles.

HORMONE   A chemical messenger in the body usually produced at one site and acting at another.

IMMUNOLOGY   A study of the defence mechanisms of the body.

METABOLISM   The chemical processes of the body.

MENOPAUSE   The period of life when menstruation normally ceases.

MONOAMINE OXIDASE   The enzyme group concerned with the breakdown of substances like noradrenaline and tyramine in the body.

NITROGLYCERINE   A substance which causes blood vessels to dilate.

ORAL CONTRACEPTION   The use of drugs taken by mouth for the purpose of preventing ovulation.

OVULATION   The expulsion of an egg cell from the ovary.

PAROXYSMAL   Recurring at intervals.

PLACEBO   An inert substance which can have no effect whatever.

RENAL THRESHOLD   The level at which glucose passes from the blood stream into the urine.

SCOTOMA   A partially blind area in the field of vision.

SEROTONIN (5HT)   A vasoactive amine found in blood.

STRESS   The response the body makes to a mental or physical challenge.

TYRAMINE   A vasoactive amine found in some cheeses.

VASOACTIVE   A substance which acts on blood vessels causing them either to constrict or dilate.

VASCULAR   Pertaining to blood vessels. Arteries carry blood from the heart. Veins carry blood to the heart.

Index